CW00459682

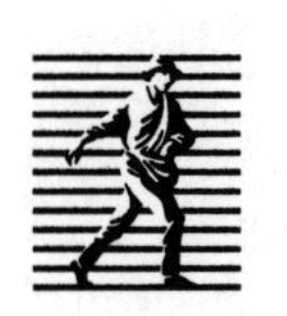

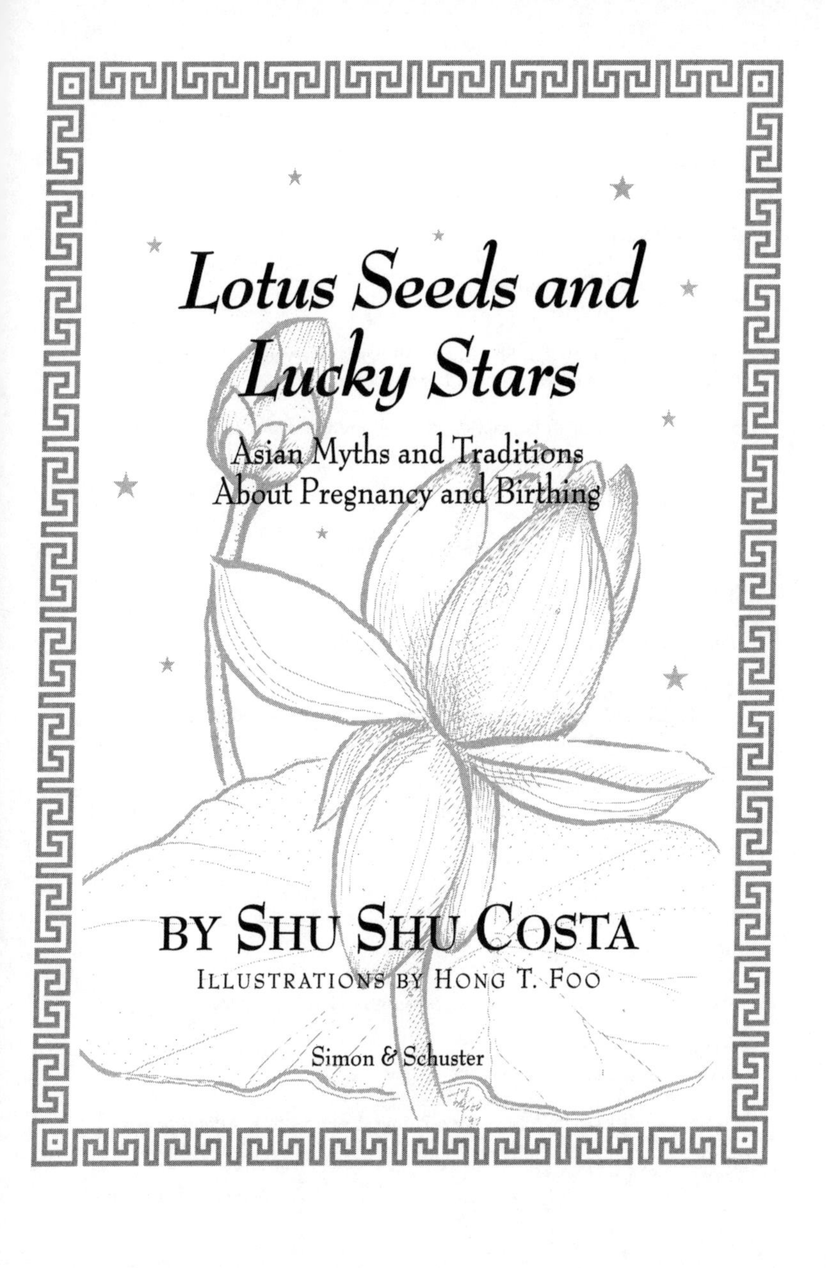

Lotus Seeds and Lucky Stars

Asian Myths and Traditions About Pregnancy and Birthing

BY SHU SHU COSTA

ILLUSTRATIONS BY HONG T. FOO

Simon & Schuster

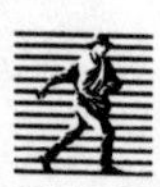

SIMON & SCHUSTER
Rockefeller Center
1230 Avenue of the Americas
New York, NY 10020

Designed by Ruth Lee

Manufactured in the United States of America

10 9 8 7 6 5 4 3 2 1

Library of Congress Cataloging-in-Publication Data

Costa, Shu Shu, date
Lotus seeds and lucky stars : Asian myths and traditions about pregnancy and birthing / by Shu Shu Costa ; illustrations by Hong T. Fu.
p. cm.
1. Birth customs—Asia. 2. Pregnancy—Asia—Folklore. 3. Childbirth—Asia—Folklore. 4. Traditional medicine—Asia. 5. Asia—Social life and customs. I. Title.
GT2465.A78C67 1998
392.1'2'095—dc21
97-53269
CIP

ISBN 0-684-84397-8

The author gratefully acknowledges permission to reprint the following:

"I grew fat . . ."
"My labor went on and on . . ."
"I cannot tell . . ."
Copyright © 1978 by Ann Warren Turner. Excerpts from *Rituals of Birth*, originally published by David McKay Co., Inc. Reprinted by permission of Curtis Brown, Ltd.

(continued on page 138)

Acknowledgments

A BOOK IS LIKE A BIRTHING; no one truly does it alone. My thanks and gratitude go first to the friends and family members all around the world who dug deep into their own family lore to share their stories. To me, these stories prove how very similar we all are, how the miracle of birth transcends culture and generation, place and time.

Next, I want to thank Annie Hughes O'Connor, for her editor's ear and her special support; Laurie Chittenden, for seeing it through; the art director and editorial staff at Simon & Schuster for their care; and my agents, Madeleine Morel and Barbara Lowenstein, for their help. They are midwives all; this book could not be born without them.

Many, many thanks to my friends and family, who fill each day with light and love. A special note of gratitude, too, goes to my father, Hong Foo, whose illustrations grace these words as they have always touched my life with beauty.

Finally, I want to thank my sons, Keith and Chad, for all that they give and for all they have taught me—you bring to my life a joy I could never have imagined. And, as always, my deepest love goes to my husband, Christopher, for his endless laughter and caring, without which nothing would be possible. With all this wealth and riches, I must have been born under the luckiest star.

O my father who begat me!
O my mother who nourished me!
Ye indulged me, ye fed me,
ye held me up, ye supported me,
out and in ye bore me in your arms.
If I would return your kindness,
it is like great Heaven, illimitable.

ANCIENT CHINESE POEM

To my parents and my sons,
with love.

Contents

Lotus Seeds and Lucky Stars

Introduction

EVERY PREGNANT WOMAN HEARS AN EARFUL of advice from the moment she announces that she is expecting. Asian-American mothers-to-be are no different—the myths just seem all the more outrageous, the wisdom all the more ancient. The source of this folklore seems deep and mysterious, pungent with the sharp smell of herbal potions, heavy with the dust of centuries of superstitions. No nailing or sawing should be done in the house where a baby is to be born, one of my aunts said to me. Nodding his head, number two uncle, the family storyteller, tells of the time he did some carpentry in front of a pregnant sow—who later gave birth to two deformed piglets. When my son was born, another aunt sent recipes for a soup with black cloud mushrooms and "drunken" chicken marinated in wine—"for clotting the blood," she told me.

Even my mother, who has lived in this country for over thirty years, started behaving strangely. Pregnancy is one of those funny times in life, like weddings or funerals, when childhood superstitions and family folklore peek like ghosts from under the most rational people. I know this side of my mother appears whenever she brings up her old aunty. Old aunty—I'm never quite sure which aunt she is—is a useful medium for my mother. It allows her to give advice that from her American side seems illogical, but from her more rooted Chinese side seems necessary.

"When I gave birth to you," my mother announced one day, "old aunty told me not to bathe for twelve days. After those twelve days were over, my first bath was full of herbs." She looked at me, hesitating. "Maybe you shouldn't take a shower for a few days after you give birth."

The idea was absolutely shocking. "Mom," I tried to reassure her, "that probably was because the water wasn't clean enough in your village."

"You never know," she said, shaking her head. She looked doubtful.

When I came home from the hospital in the middle of summer, my mother didn't let me drink anything cold, but insisted I drink hot tea boiled with ginger and roasted rice, "to bring my heat back." Other special foods were cooked and prepared to preserve my "heat" and keep away the "cold." For two weeks, I was not to do anything but rest and care for my new son—the Chinese call this "sitting for a month." Her behavior, as inexplicable as it seemed at times, comforted the two of us. I am sure her mother and her old aunty, in a different place and a different time, did the same things for her.

The myths and stories of pregnancy and childbirth collected here come from mothers and aunties and grandmothers in this country and throughout Asia. Like my mother's advice, they come from places where wisdom was passed on from generation to generation, mother to daughter, by word of mouth. Much of the advice seems humorous in this modern day and modern country. In Japan, a pregnant woman never looks at fire, so the baby is not born with scars. In Korea, chicken is avoided, so the baby is not born with "chicken skin."

Lotus Seeds and Lucky Stars will give voice to these Asian mothers and their "older aunties," to their myths and superstitions, their wisdom and their love. Folklore dealing with conception, foretelling the sex of the child, and caring for the unborn baby will be retold. Home remedies from Asia will be shared, exotic herbal potions to cleanse the mother and smooth her complexion, foul-tasting concoctions to nourish the baby, foods that heal and soothe. Rituals that welcome the new child, protect the baby and mother from evil spirits, assure them both a place in society, or even get the mother back in shape, will be described. I hope you will enjoy these tales and pass them on to your own friends and relatives.

Oddly enough, there are times, too, when the old aunty has proved her wisdom. I've come across pregnancy myths that do ring true, even to our Western ears. One myth from Southeast Asia warns a pregnant woman to sleep on her side, not her back—a notion written off by the anthropologist who noted it in the 1960s. These days, doctors advise women to do just that; sleeping on the back, research has found, puts pressure on the baby's blood supply.

Perhaps I shouldn't have taken that shower after all.

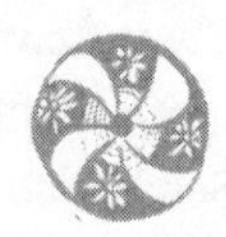

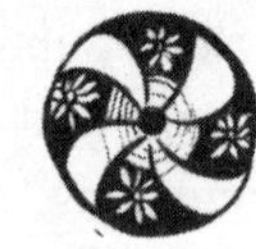

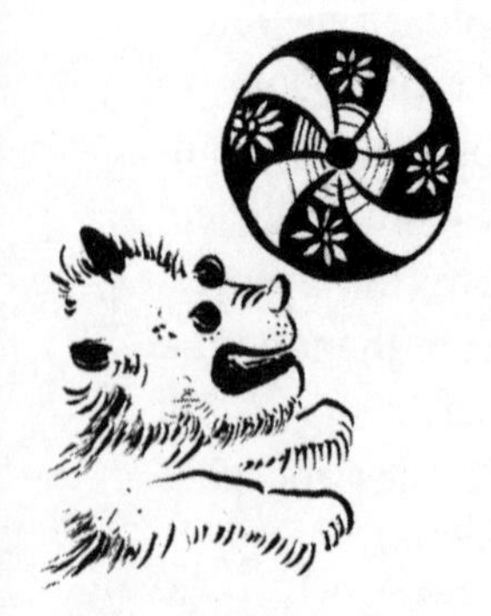

1

Getting Pregnant: Blessings, Offerings, and Prayers

Arm in arm,
my mother and father
searched a cavern
and found a gold-lit pond.

Lots of lotuses
were covering it,
dewdrops
on curling leaves.

I, a light-
hearted girl,
was born.

A MODERN KOREAN BIRTH DREAM

EVERY WOMAN, THE CHINESE BELIEVE, has a flowering tree growing in the unseen world of spirits and gods. For some, the tree is filled with red flowers, for boys. For some, the flowers are white, for girls. For still others, the tree is lifeless, barren. Only a wise fortune teller can peer into the shadows of that world and tell if you are to be blessed with offspring or cursed—as women were in ancient Asia—forever.

In older times, having children was a sacred duty. It was the very reason for marriage, to create another generation to pay respects to the ancestors, to carry on the family name with honor. A son could kowtow before the ancestors, sweep their graves, and care for his parents into their old age. A daughter could be married into a family rich with wealth or prestige, raising her own family's social standing. Producing children was so important that the Chinese word for "good," *hao,* is created from two characters, one for "woman" or "mother," and the other for "children." And in Japan, as recently as fifty years ago, a wife was not placed on her husband's official registry until she produced a baby boy.

The importance of children, combined with the deep mystery of conception, created fanciful myths and rituals that betray some of the anxiety and fascination in this most magical time. Perhaps you've heard some of them firsthand, from older relatives waiting for that grandchild, from mothers who believe in birth dreams, from fathers sharing the myths of the man chopping trees on the moon. Symbolic wedding gifts, elaborate doll offerings, potent aphrodisiacs—these were the ways our ancestors could beseech the gods who watched over them for the blessing of a child. For whatever the stresses placed on a new bride by the family, whatever offering or wish you use to bring about a child, whatever way you believe a baby is created, in the end, the joy of new life is universal, transcending time or place or culture.

Gifts and Offerings for the Blessing of a Child

My mother began talking of grandchildren long before my wedding date was actually set. A twinkle would appear in her eye, and she would exclaim, "I can't wait to be a grandmother!" Westerners might view this kind of talk as parental pressure. For me, this was just my mother's Asian side peeking out, undaunted by thirty years of Western concepts of what may be "politically correct" to say to an adult child.

I'm sure she would be surprised that every parent, Asian or Western, doesn't act that way. In Asia, talk of children begins as soon as a wedding is announced, if not before. Having children is so important; why be subtle? Traditional wedding gifts, for example, are heavy with symbolism relating to children. In China—and even today among Chinese-Americans—brides are given a set of chopsticks with their dowry, the word for chopsticks, *fai ji,* sounding like "fast boy." Engagement gifts of pomegranates—the countless sections symbolizing many sons—and a deer horn, an aphrodisiac, are yet another wish for children. At the traditional tea ceremony, where the bride and groom are formally introduced to their families, the sweet offering is made with dried lotus seeds, their name, *lian zi,* sounding like the phrase "successive sons." Lotus seeds are also traditionally served for dessert at the wedding banquet.

A Japanese bride-to-be is given a special envelope of *konbu,* a seaweed, with her engagement gifts. The word *konbu* can also mean "child-bearing woman." *Konbu* is also a popular garnish or ingredient in the Japanese wedding banquet. Salted herring roe, the eggs, representing children, of course, is also popular. Finally, a traditional wedding cake, *komochi manjyu,* a large mounded pastry filled with sweetened bean paste in five colors, symbolizes many offspring.

In Kulawi, Indonesia, brass charms of naked men and women were once thought to enhance fertility. These magical charms were carried by just-married women, displayed in the homes of newlyweds or weighed in during marriage negotiations. They were thought to protect a couple from evil.

The Korean wedding ceremony is highlighted by the ritual throwing of dates and chestnuts. Following the *p'yebaek* ceremony, in which the bride pays her respects to her new family, her new in-laws toss dates and chestnuts—symbols of children—for her to catch in her large *hanbok,* the wedding skirt. The more she catches with her traditional dress, the more children she will be blessed with. (You can be sure her in-laws aim well!) Earlier, at the *kunbere* wedding ceremony, a hen with a symbolic chestnut in its mouth graced the offerings table.

Not surprisingly, America inherited from Asia the custom of throwing rice—symbol of life and fertility—at the wedding couple.

The Chinese believe that there are good and bad times to conceive. The male partner should be thirty years old, a time when he is at his physical peak. The woman should be twenty, a time when she is full of *qi* (loosely translated as "life force" or "energy"), blood, and *jing* (the body's physical essence, responsible for the creation of new life). Timing the act of procreation is also important. According to traditional Chinese medicine, conception must be avoided:

at noon, or the child will vomit a lot;
at midnight, or the child will be deaf and/or mute;
during a solar eclipse, or the child will be weak;
during a thunder and lightning storm, or the child will be insane;
during a lunar eclipse, or both mother and child will have bad luck;
during the winter or summer solstice, or both mother and child will suffer;
during the full moon, or the child will suffer eye diseases;
while intoxicated or on a full stomach, or the child will have a tendency toward insanity, carbuncles, or piles.

Other times to avoid conception are while either partner is suffering from a skin disease; during menstruation;

while in mourning; 100 days after a hot or warm disease; or while in distress or shock.

The best time to conceive is after midnight between three and five A.M., a time when yin and yang are well balanced. A child created at this time is believed to be intelligent, energetic, relaxed, and beautiful.

Symbols and traditions aside, you can't have a baby without firing up the libido. In the old wives' chemistry books of Asia, three foods are guaranteed to make men wild for sex: dog (Korea), snakes (Cantonese), and the brains of live monkeys (Thailand). Of course, for today's Asian-Americans, whose palate and supermarket may not support live monkey brains, oysters and asparagus might do just fine.

Yet, if all those wedding gifts and aphrodisiacs don't work, and you haven't conceived within the next year, your parents may pull out a new bag of tricks. In older times, a new wife's worst nightmare was to be barren. After a grace period of a few years, she might be sent home in disgrace, or her husband might bring home another wife or a concubine. To prevent this shame, a bride's parents sent a special care package on a lucky day between the fifth and fourteenth day of the first month of the year. In it was a paper lantern with the image of Kuan Yin, the Goddess of Mercy and a sort of Buddhist Virgin Mary, often depicted with a child in her arms. Rice cakes, oranges, garlic, and oysters in an earthenware vessel round out the package.

Each item has a special meaning: The name of the cakes, or *kao,* sounds like the word for "elder brother," implying that you will have more than one son. The word for oysters, *tieh,* sounds like "younger brother"; the earthen vessel, *kou,* sounds like the word for "to come." Oranges, *chi,* sound like "speedy," and garlic, *saung kiang,* sounds like "grandchildren and children." All in all, the message is clear: May you have many sons *soon.*

If yet another year passes, the parents send yet another lantern, this one with the inscription "The child seated in the tub"—a reference to the wooden tub that was once commonly used to receive babies after birth. If, after the third year, there is no baby in sight, an orange-shaped lantern and a stick of sugarcane is sent. The sugarcane is sectioned like a piece of bamboo, the many sections implying, again, many sons. The flowers of the rape with its abundant seeds hint at the same, while the name for bean curd, *tao hou,* sounds like the words "sure to have."

Another, perhaps more modern gift to give a couple trying to conceive is a scroll or silk hanging of the famous picture of "one hundred infants." This design of children in olden-day court life alludes to the golden era of Yao and Shun, when, so the tale goes, the people of China were so prosperous that they felt as "lighthearted as children." There are actually only ninety-nine children in the piece, a reference to Wen Wang, Duke of Chou, 1231–1135 B.C., who had ninety-nine children of his own and adopted one more, a child he found in a field after a thunderstorm.

Still No Baby? Try Begging the Gods

Babies, so the myths go, come from the gods, who luckily can be beseeched by special offerings and extraordinary efforts. Thousands of pilgrims—mostly women, but some men—still make the trip to Mount Tai in the Shandong province of northern China to ask the goddesses for a child. Mount Tai is the most important of the five sacred peaks of Taoism. As the easternmost peak, the first to touch the dawn of the sun, it is viewed as a point where life begins. (Intriguingly, it is also seen as the place where life ends—at its base is the entrance to the Chinese hell.)

The most popular deity in residence on Mount Tai is the Goddess of Mount Tai, Taishan Niangniang, also called Bixia Yuanjin. Her specialty is providing children, especially male heirs. She is assisted in her duties by a group of lower-ranking goddesses, including the Eye Goddess (Yan'guang Niangniang), the Goddess of Posterity and Conception (Zisun Niangniang), the Delivers Children Goddess (Songzi Niangniang), the Goddess who Determines Birth Date (Zhusheng Niangniang), the Midwife Goddess (Cuisheng Niangniang), the Goddess of Breastfeeding (Naimu Niangniang), and the Protectress of Little Children (Yinmeng Niangniang).

The best time of the year to pray to the Goddess of

Mount Tai is on her birthday, which falls at different times of the year, depending on where you live: In Shandong, it falls on the fifteenth day of the third lunar month. In Beijing and Tianjin, it falls on the eighteenth day of the fourth lunar month. If you can't make the arduous journey to Mount Tai, a number of smaller temples around China will suffice.

If, however, you live in America, and can't make the trip to China, you might try this fertility rite at home. The most important ritual for praying to any of the goddesses is called *shuan wawa,* "tying a baby doll." A piece of red string or yarn is tied around the neck of a baby doll, and the doll is placed on the altar of the temple or shrine. Tying the red string secures the baby's spirit to the womb of the mother. In other cases, a woman may wrap a red cloth very tightly around the doll and place it on the altar. She then prays to the goddess for a child, using incense and "spirit money" and offering such delicacies as homemade food or hand-embroidered shoes. After kowtowing three times, she takes the doll home and places it on or next to her bed. For the ambitious, red cloth can also be purchased from enterprising monks at the top of Mount Tai, to be placed on the bed of the couple trying to conceive. It is hoped that the blessed cloth will pass on some of the goddess's powers of conception.

Japanese women also use dolls to encourage the spirits of conception. The old women of a village visit the home of a woman wanting a child. There, with the help of the woman wishing to conceive, they mime the whole process of labor and delivery. At the final push, as serious as any midwife, they triumphantly hold up the doll.

Asian gods come in all shapes and sizes. In Korea, women can be found praying to waterfalls, to phallic or vulva-shaped stones, or kneeling before an image of the Seven Stars (Big Dipper) Spirit, Ch'ilsong, or the Mountain God, Sanshin, to ask for the birth of a child. Many pray for a hundred days—the number being the symbol of perfection—or until the gods answer them in their dreams.

One Korean businessman relates this dream, described to him by his mother:

> My mother had been married for eight years, but wasn't able to bear any children. Her parents-in-law scolded her every day because she hadn't given birth to a son. She prayed at many shrines, and in particular, before one penis-shaped stone, dedicated to the Seven Stars god.
>
> Every morning before dawn, she would get up and wash her hair and body in clear water. Shc would leave the house, without having eaten anything, about five A.M., and walk through the countryside for about two hours to the stone, where she would pray, for it was believed that the god came down into that stone and gave the spirit of a son to a faithful woman. She would continue praying all day long and return home about ten P.M.

> She kept doing this for one hundred days, even in the cold winter, until finally, at home, she had a dream:
>
> She was coming home from her daily routine of prayer when a big yellow snake crossed the road in front of her. She woke up, and soon found that she had indeed conceived. I was that child, her son.

The full moon, which hangs heavy in the harvest season sky, figures in two myths from Asia: In old Korea, people believed that the harvest moon was a spirit who could fertilize a woman's womb. On the night of the full moon, virgins dressed in flowing white dresses danced in spirals and sang "Kanggang suwollae," hoping to one day be blessed with a child.

In Chinese legend, the rogue Wu-Gang, once from Hsi-Ho in western China, has been trying for centuries to cut down the cassia tree that grows on the moon. The cassia tree is very large, and its leaves are always green. How Wu-Gang got to the moon, nobody knows. Some say he escaped there after killing someone; others say it was the only place to go after he lost everything to his gambling debts; yet another tale has him banished to the moon by an angry Jade Emperor. Night after night, he tries to cut down this mighty tree, shaking it to its core. Yet, every time he manages to make an ax cut, the tree miraculously heals itself.

On the day of the midautumn festival, the fifteenth day of the eighth moon, families gather to celebrate the harvest, to eat mooncakes, and to watch the full moon, the perfect circle a symbol of family harmony. Legend has it that, on this night, a woman who swallows one of the cassia leaves that has fallen to earth will become pregnant.

If you can't find a cassia leaf, you might try another goddess, Kuan Yin. This goddess of mercy—the name Kuan Yin literally means "Hear the cries," a reference to the many prayers she answers—is often depicted dressed in beautiful, white flowing robes and holding a child. Her help is sought in all types of problems, but she is especially sensitive to wishes for children. Villagers in southern China pray to her on the nineteenth day of the second, sixth, and ninth moons.

The story of Kuan Yin goes like this: According to legend, Kuan Yin was the daughter of a Chou dynasty sovereign who longed to be a Buddhist nun. Her father was so upset by his daughter's refusal to marry that he subjected her to humiliating tasks at the convent in the hope that she would recant. When that failed, he ordered her to be put to death for disobedience. The kind executioner, however, broke the sword that was to kill her into a thousand pieces. Foiled again, her father ordered her to be strangled.

This time, Kuan Yin died and went to hell. But upon the arrival of this pure soul, the flames were quenched and flowers began to bloom. The presiding officer of hell, Yama, was so dismayed that he sent her back to life again, her body carried in the fragrant heart of a lotus flower. Kuan Yin lived her life on a small island until, one day, she heard that her father had become ill. In the ultimate act of filial piety, she cut the flesh from her arm so that it might be made into medicine for a cure. His life was saved, and Kuan Yin was forgiven. Her tender spirit and great devotion to family make her a popular choice for worshipers who pray for children.

Where Do Babies Come From?

What could be more mythical than conception? Even now, creating a baby seems to be pure magic. But before the days of blood tests and ovulation kits, where babies come from was anybody's guess. In rural Malaysia, the baby's life is thought to begin in the brain of the father. For forty days, the baby's soul slowly travels down from the head to the heart and finally out the penis, where it enters the mother. Some men even remember having had cravings for foods before their wives became pregnant!

With this image of conception, the baby inherits the father's rationality and emotions—important in this patrilineal society. The sex of the baby, they believe, is also determined in the father's brain, but it can be changed through prayer.

The idea that the baby's spirit is not fixed at the moment of conception is also found in the villages of Thailand. It is believed that the soul of the child, the *khwan,* flies into the womb during sex to create the fetus. But that soul may not stay for long. It is believed that several souls of obscure origin—and unknown worth—drift in and out of the woman's body until one finally takes up residence. Mothers pray that their baby will inherit a divine soul, not the soul of a criminal.

Not all babies are conceived after intercourse: Legend has it that Confucius's mother became pregnant with him after she stepped in the footsteps of a unicorn. Momotaro, the magical child who slew Japan's monstrous *oni* with the help of a few gods, was born inside a beautiful golden peach.

No matter how a baby is created, Asians believe the moment of conception is so powerful that many mothers experience a profound dream about their unborn child around that time. Called *t'aemong* (Korean) or *t'aimeng* (Chinese), these birth dreams foretell the sex of the child or the future personality or success of the baby. One explanation for these dreams is this: The Koreans believe that three gods coexist in each person and create these vivid images in our subconscious—the Heaven god, the Earth god, and the Man god. When a mother experiences a *t'aemong*, the image she is seeing is the Man god of her unborn child, preparing her for what is to come.

In these dreams, mothers may also get a glimpse of the "birth grandmother" who delivers the child from the gods to the mother's womb. Like the Western stork who flies around the world delivering children, this white-haired Samshin Halmoni or "womb-spirit grandmother" may appear in an expectant woman's dream bearing a gift, which sometimes symbolizes the sex of the child. Some believe this grandmother cares for the child for forty-nine days after birth, before retiring to the heavens. Others believe she is the baby's god, appearing in the mother's dreams four or five times, and staying until a hundred days after the birth of a child. For many families, one particular heavenly messenger returns again and again over generations—a personal "stork."

The Chinese also believe in a stork, of sorts. They believe a celestial fairy rides atop a majestic unicorn delivering babies to be reborn on earth. This fairy decides where and when purified Buddhist souls will be reincarnated.

With the blessing of the celestial fairy, your mythical tree is in full bloom. The next nine months will be filled with birth dreams of your own, dreams of your future child, dreams of your new role as parent. For our grandmothers and great-grandmothers, pregnancy was a time to relax, a time when an expectant mother's every wish and desire were met. It was also a time of worry; myths and legends tell of witches and mischievious spirits who lurk in dark corners waiting to steal unborn babies. Truth be told, all women, no matter what the culture or what the age, do a little bit of both. Cherish these moments as you cherish the springtime: The tree is in bloom; the harvest is soon to come.

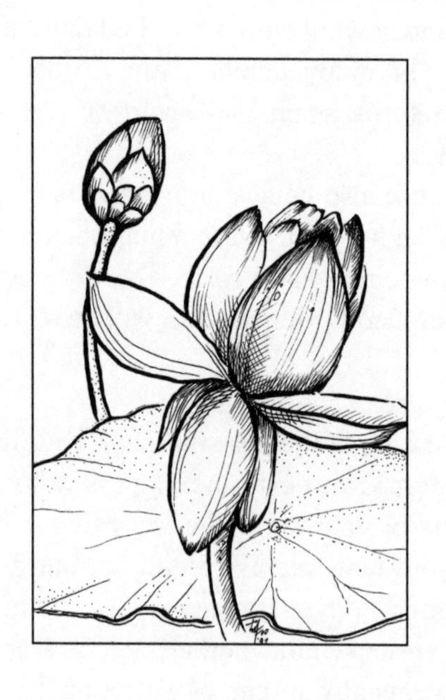

2

Pregnancy Myths: Reading Poetry and Avoiding Knives

> *A pregnant woman carries with her the finest piece of jade. She should enjoy all things, look at fine pictures, and be attended by handsome servants.*
>
> ADMONITIONS TO LADIES,
>
> ASIAN MEDICAL GUIDE FOR WOMEN

WHEN YOU ARE A NEW MOTHER-TO-BE, your whole life changes. While you probably don't have many handsome servants, still, you grab a piece of fruit instead of a cookie, catch a little catnap, if you can, and take your prenatal vitamin religiously. In Asia, even today, a pregnant woman takes her care one step further. As her ancestors did before her, she guards her mind and thoughts, as well as her actions. It is believed that her whole being—her physical, mental, and moral states, everything she sees, everything she does—will influence the unborn child. She is urged to read good poetry and think lofty thoughts, to never sit on a mat that is not straight or look at clashing colors. She should never gossip, never laugh loudly, and never lose her temper. She should avoid situations in which she might be fearful or anxious. Before she sleeps, she must listen to beautiful stories, and use only refined language. Sex is strictly forbidden throughout the entire pregnancy. If she does all this, her child will be born perfect.

Rituals of Birth, a collection by Ann Warren Turner of women's thoughts on childbirth from various cultures, describes how expectant mothers in old China were pampered in every way. The household's attention was focused on the creator of the future son. For traditional women, cut off from their families and residing in the home of their in-laws, the time period was one to be savored.

> I grew fat like the moon in the season of silkworms. And as moths are drawn to the moon, so the women of our house fluttered around me. Even my bronze-tongued mother-in-law was careful of me during that time. What could she do for "her Ling"? Did I desire volumes of fine poetry or the blind storyteller down the street? I said "yes" to all her suggestions and basked in the rare attention. I listened to beautiful poetry and stories; delicate pictures were hung in my room, and my clothes were of brightly colored silk. All these things would create good influences around the baby. No bad words could reach my ears, no ugly sights offend me, no bad food be given to me.

Fetal education, as this two-thousand-year-old theory is called, takes many different forms across Asia. In Korea, for example, it is called *tae kyo,* "womb education." "If I seemed harried," says one Korean-American, "my grandmother would scold, '*Ma um ul chong-hi kajora*' or 'Always keep yourself in peace.'" In Asian thinking, the mind and the body are inseparable, an idea that is beginning to take root in the West. The explanation of the effect of the heart on the baby gets a little bit fuzzy, however. Traditional Chinese medical books explain that the spirit or mind resides in the heart, which is connected by an important internal channel to the uterus. Anything that affects a woman's mind therefore affects the heart, which has a direct connection to the baby in the uterus. Therefore, positive, uplifting emotions can only have a positive effect on the development of the child.

Superstition? Perhaps. True or not, Western researchers are finding that some forms of fetal education are valid. By the end of the second trimester, an unborn child can detect light, hear sounds, and become aware of things happening near her mother's body. Some pregnant women listen to Mozart every day with the hope that their children may become music lovers or better mathematicians. (A friend in Japan attended a performance of the local symphony orchestra presented specifically for pregnant women. It was, not surprisingly, packed.) Other women read to their bellies, hoping that the child will develop a love for literature. One concert pianist, who spent six months rehearsing one particular piece while she was pregnant, claims that the piece still soothes her crying newborn. If outside influences can affect an unborn child, perhaps the effect of the mother's emotions is the next logical step.

Of course, the flip and funny side of this mother/child connection is the many myths that pregnant women hear every day. Eating too many lemons or pickles leads to a child with a sour disposition. Or lifting your hands above your head will cause the umbilical cord to wrap around the baby's neck. Asian-Americans hear all these ideas and more from solicitous mothers and aunts. The passing of time and the strangeness of the culture makes them perhaps all the more outrageous. Some of the so-called advice has been passed down since the days of Confucius; a few ring true, even to our Western ears. Judge for yourself, and beware!

Pregnancy Taboos for Mothers-to-Be

Of Food

- If you eat a lot of chicken, your baby will be born with loose "chicken skin" (Korea).
- If you eat crab, your baby will bite a lot (Korea).
- If you eat bananas, you will have a dull, lazy child (Philippines), or the baby will have a lot of gas (Malaysia).
- If your food is poorly cut or mashed, your child will have a careless disposition (China).

- If you eat light-colored food, the baby will have a fair complexion (China).
- If you eat sour foods, you'll have a miscarriage. Avoid fatty and spicy foods, too (Japan).
- Avoid lamb and mutton, because they're not healthy for the baby (Malaysia).

Of Behavior:

- If you look at an unattractive person, your baby will be born ugly (Taiwan).
- If you look at ugly pictures, your baby will be born ugly (Philippines).
- If you look at pretty pictures, your baby will be pretty (China).
- If you look at fire, your baby will be born with scars (Japan).
- If you mock or speak poorly of others, your baby will be born with those characteristics (Malaysia).
- No construction work should be done in the house. Cutting, sawing, nailing, and hammering may lead to an abortion or cause deformities in the fetus (China and Malaysia) or lead to a difficult labor (Philippines).
- Loud noises such as those caused by hammering and drilling will cause deformities as well (Taiwan).
- Don't move the furniture, especially the bed, for the same reason (Malaysia).
- Cutting or sewing in bed will harm the baby's internal organs (Taiwan).
- Don't lift anything heavy—your bones are too fragile (Korea).

- Heavy lifting or raising your hands above your head will lead to a miscarriage (China).
- Don't reach for things above your head (Japan) or wear a scarf around your neck (Philippines). The umbilical cord could wrap around the baby's neck.
- Never lie on your back (China).
- Sitting on stairs will lead to arrested labor (Philippines).
- No sex, obscene noises, or pornography (China).
- Never wear miniskirts. Cold temperatures are not good for the baby and may cause a miscarriage (Japan).
- Never attend funerals. Mothers involved in beginning a life should not be associated with the end of life (China).

Pregnancy Taboos for the Father-to-Be

Amazingly enough, in some countries, fathers are also required to be on their best behavior when their wives are pregnant. Here are some wives' tales directed just at fathers.

- Tying knots will lead to a difficult labor for your wife (Philippines).
- Do not cut your hair until the baby is born (Malaysia).
- No sitting in doorsteps. The symbolic "blocking of the birth canal" will lead to a hard labor (Malaysia).
- Do not harm anybody or any creature (Malaysia).
- Do not have sexual relations with your wife throughout her pregnancy (China).

Watching over Mother-to-Be and Baby, Too

In America, we watch what we eat, try to exercise, and hope that our pregnancy is successful. Our grandmothers, in addition to paying attention to all that was taboo, had different, more serious, concerns: For centuries, Asian mothers-to-be fought hard to keep the evil spirits from taking their unborn babies. Living in a world where the gods—the good, bad, and merely mischievious—were as close as your next-door neighbor, women held a healthy respect for these otherworldly powers. In the Philippines, families lit fires made with *suwa* or *baungon* leaves under their homes so witches would not suck the blood of the expectant mother. And in Malaysia, mothers-to-be would forgo an afternoon nap, for fear that an evil spirit would catch them unawares and snatch the baby away.

In China, women placed long, sharp knives on their beds to frighten away evil spirits who might come in the night. The shape of a pair of scissors was cut from paper and pinned to the bed curtains, and tiger skins were hung over the bed. Fierce-looking objects and the forms of other wild animals cut from paper were put around the room and on the windows to protect the mother from these spirits.

When the mother-to-be ventured out, a smelly fishing net was placed over her sedan chair. Priests used such nets to catch demons, so it was believed that this would also discourage any spirits from harming the mother.

During the fifth month, women held a special ceremony to thank the goddess—perhaps the Goddess of Mount Tai or Kuan Yin—for the good health of the fetus. With offerings of homemade food, heady incense, and mock money or spirit money, they'd pray for the goddess's continued protection and for an easy delivery.

The Japanese also have a ritual for the fifth month of pregnancy. A strip of cotton, called *iwata-obi* or *sarashi,* is tied around the expectant mother's waist, just below her extended belly. Depending on the village or family, the belt is made from the father's loincloth, given by the parents, or borrowed from the shrine whose god helps with childbirth. Most are white, with the words *an zan,* meaning safety, written on them. Measuring 13 inches by 5 yards, the material is folded in half and secured tightly at both ends, leaving some slack in the middle. For practical purposes, the belt provides warmth for the abdomen and also helps women carry the baby.

A Shinto ceremony, always held on the day of the dog, is performed when the belt is put in place. Some *iwata-obi* also sport the print of a dog. Why the dog? Because dogs, lucky things, are supposed to have easy births.

Preparing for Baby's Arrival

In the West, the mother-to-be spends a good deal of time preparing for her baby's arrival. That might mean preparing the nursery, buying baby clothes, carriages, and cribs, or attending showers given by friends and family.

My mother was a bit hesistant to throw me a baby shower. In China, it is considered unlucky to have a party for the baby before the little one actually arrives. Instead, baby's big day comes one month after the child is born. In Japan, they are more optimistic; a birth is celebrated on the seventh day, when relatives and friends bring gifts for mother and child. In Korea, an elaborate party is thrown after a hundred days. Before that time, the parents dare not publicly celebrate the birth; the child might be too weak to survive. (Most celebrations are held after the baby's birth. See chapter 7 for rituals and traditions that celebrate the newborn child.)

One tradition takes place *before* the birth. In China, the mother-to-be's own mother is responsible for the entire layette. One month before delivery, she sends a package of clothing, mostly for her expectant daughter, called *tsui shen,* "hastening the delivery." The only item for the baby is a soft white cloth in which to wrap the newborn. Three days after the baby is born, the new grandmother comes to visit, bringing all the newborn's clothes and any equipment needed. The more wealthy the family, the more elaborate the layette. Often a family will spend a huge sum for a layette to enhance their daughter's prestige with her in-laws.

Naming the Baby

In the West, couples begin discussing names for the baby before the baby is born. You wouldn't dream of doing such a thing in the East. In China, babies are first given false names to scare away any evil spirits who might wish to steal them away. Called "milk names," these temporary monikers are given at the one-month birthday. They often refer to an animal, such as "Little Cat" or "Little Puppy," to try to fool the spirits into thinking the child is an animal and not worth taking. Or they choose adjectives such as "ugly" or "stupid," to convince the mischievious gods that the child is not worth taking.

My friend, a new mother, discovered this firsthand while proudly showing off her newborn to an older family friend. "What an ugly baby," said the woman to my friend, who looked at her in shock. Ugly? The older woman smiled sweetly and handed the baby back. It's customary, she explained, to say only bad things about a baby when it is first born, so the evil spirits will avoid taking the child.

Once the child is older, it is given a real name. The Chinese sometimes have four or five names—one for childhood, one when they enter school, another after graduation, and another entering business. Often, a new name is given even after death.

As in all cultures, names have special significance. Asians believe that your name can bring good luck or bad luck throughout your life. Some families even consult fortune-tellers for an appropriate name! In Japan, children are named after departed parents. The Japanese believe that when people die, their souls await reincarnation belowground. These souls reenter the world through the bodies of newborn babies.

How do you know which ancestor has returned? One way is to hold the baby up in the air when he or she cries. The names of departed ancestors are repeated until the baby stops crying. When the baby is calm, the right ancestor has been named.

The Chinese and Koreans also pay homage to family ties by using generational names, names common to one particular generation. My family did just that, naming all my female cousins Phaik and all male cousins Kean. For outsiders, these names show which family you belong to; for family members, they place you among the hierarchy. The names of the males of my family hold an even greater legacy: The generational names join together to form a poem that is inscribed on a rock at the family village in China. All told, we've recorded twenty-four generations of the Foo family, all linked by this poem. As the various branches of the family have spread, each has chosen to continue the poem, sometimes adding lines to describe its part of the family history.

Most likely, your family has some naming traditions as well, perhaps a legacy to follow or modify as you choose. My husband and I chose to honor both sides of our family, naming our son after my husband's father, Keith. His middle name, Yeh, is the next generational name in my family. Thus he has the best of both worlds. Other families might choose a fully Asian name and another Western name for their children, or one or the other. You may want to ask a family member if your family has any naming traditions. Or, since this is a start of a new generation, perhaps you may want to create a tradition of your own.

If you're worried that the name you've chosen is not the best one for your child, try this trick, used by the villagers of Malaysia: The midwife recites a series of potential names while dropping rice grains into a glass of water. The wrong name causes the rice to drop to the bottom. Three floating rice grains mean you have chosen the correct name.

✧ ✧ ✧

Myths are tricky things. With one side of our head we laugh at how outrageous they sound. On the other hand, as my Korean-American friend pointed out, they've been around for thousands of years. "Surely there must be something to them," she says. Is there? If not, why are so many so similar to each other? Western science is finding secrets hidden in many Asian herbal remedies—could there be wisdom hidden in Asian old wives' tales?

The other day, as I reached both hands over my head, doing some prenatal exercises, these thoughts raced through my head. Guiltily, I lowered my hands and put them instinctively over my belly. My mother's clear and gentle voice, probably layered with generations of mothers' voices, came into my head. "You never know," she said. "You never know."

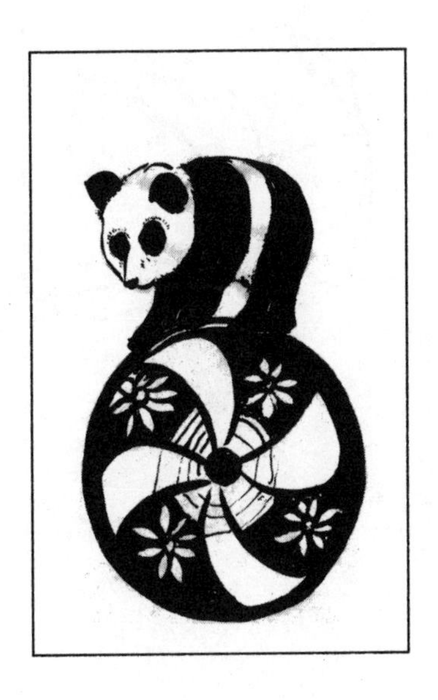

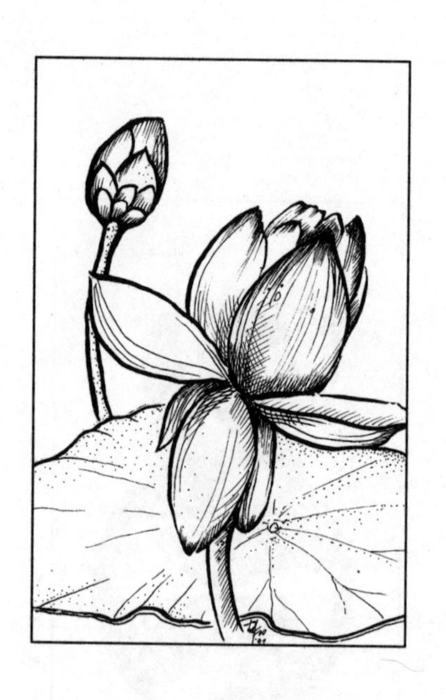

3

Herbal Potions, Ancient Medical Advice, and Home Remedies

Young's Remedy for Morning Sickness

Ginger Tea:
¼ pound of ginger steeped in
boiling water. Sugar to taste.

NATURE LETS YOU KNOW RIGHT AWAY when you're pregnant. One morning you feel fine, the next you can't stand the smell of coffee. Throughout the nine months, you are bound to feel the discomfort of carrying twenty-five to thirty-five extra pounds of weight, twelve of which have pushed your other organs up into your ribs and, through the last six months, kick *hard*.

For most of these problems, there are few solutions. Modern medicine can cause all sorts of side effects damaging to a growing fetus. Practitioners of Chinese medicine, however, say they can alleviate some of the discomforts of pregnancy. In addition, there are always old auntie's many home remedies to relieve the headaches, backaches, and stomach problems common in pregnancy.

Chinese medicine has been practiced for thousands of

years. The herbal remedies of other Asian cultures are all based on classical Chinese medicine. To the Westerner, its theories seem very mysterious and downright unscientific. But as one modern writer put it, Eastern and Western medicine are merely two different, but no less valid, maps of the same place. More and more, Western doctors are beginning to acknowledge the validity of such practices as acupuncture. And Americans now spend millions each year on herbal concoctions, many of which come from the East.

When I was growing up, my parents' medicine chest was filled with strange-smelling, foul-tasting herbal remedies. Instead of Benadryl for insect bites, there was *ipoh ewe,* a clear liquid that burned like a tiny fire and smelled of strong camphor. Instead of Pepto-Bismol, there were *po chai* pills, hundreds of tiny dark-red pills that felt like candy going down your throat. For menstrual cramps, there was a bitter brown powder that, when mixed with a tablespoon of water, tasted and smelled like mud from the bottom of your shoe. (Grape flavor has not yet hit Asian medicines.)

My mother has been trying to convince me of their validity for years. And for years, I've taken her advice with a grain of salt. If the *po chai* pills didn't work—my Western husband, by the way, swears by them—I had a bottle of Pepto-Bismol as a backup. I couldn't bear the taste of the stuff for cramps, so I invested in Midol early. But as more scientific research is done on these centuries-old remedies, I'm starting to change my mind. Just a bit.

The home remedies and medical advice described here are by no means a prescription. I'm not a doctor, and you should never take any remedy, herbal or otherwise, without consulting yours first. Much of the advice I've collected from family, friends, and medical literature is mostly common sense. Many remedies, as is the case in most Asian cultures, are food based. Some of them, like the ginger tea, are wonderfully soothing. Some, like the balance of yin and yang, hot and cold foods, are a bit mysterious. Others, like the blood of carp, are only for the brave and the true believers. Perhaps, among these anodynes, is one your grandmother has been telling you about for years. Or maybe one remedy will help in just the right way. Personally, I'll stick to the ginger tea.

Herbal Potions, Ancient Remedies

In America, one of the first medicines prescribed by doctors for pregnant women is the prenatal vitamin. Mine is very fancy; it's even "vanilla-scented" to improve the flavor for the two and a half seconds you have it in your mouth.

In contrast to my pleasant-tasting pill, my pregnant cousin in Malaysia had to drink a special herbal concoction called *chap jee thai por* that her mother bought from the local Chinese drugstore. Literally, that means "drink to help maintain the fetus." Herbs were boiled in three and a half bowls of water that condensed into one, bitter, horrible-tasting cup of tea she drank once a week until the middle of her pregnancy. Another potion, *chap sar thai por,* nourishes the fetus for the second half of the pregnancy—and it doesn't taste much better.

There are other potions sold by the local Chinese drugstore in Malaysia you can try: *tau foo fa,* for example, gives the mother a beautiful complexion. *Chuan lian* is taken just before delivery to prevent the child from having boils. In fact, Chinese medicine has a whole host of remedies for various pregnancy ailments. Unlike Western medicine, Chinese medicine seeks to treat "patterns of disharmony," the specific symptoms unique to each patient. Western medicine focuses on diagnosing a disease and then prescribing the standard medicine. Because the Chinese remedy is individualized—so the theory goes—there are fewer side effects. Chinese medical practitioners can prescribe herbal remedies for standard pregnancy annoyances such as nausea and vomiting, edema, coughs, and diarrhea. They also believe they can help more serious ailments, such as high blood pressure, and can deal with ectopic pregnancies.

What to Expect Month by Month, Chinese-Style

Along with medicines to help the mother-to-be and nourish the fetus, Chinese classical medicine offers advice on the behavior and lifestyle of the mother. Nothing concerns a pregnant woman more than the development of her unborn child. We eat right, avoid preservatives, and worry incessantly about our child's health. Science tells us day by day, month by month, what to expect: the organs begin to form in the first month, the hair in the fifth. Sun Simiao, a famous Chinese doctor of the Tang Dynasty, A.D. 618 to 907, made his own calculations. It's interesting to note that his advice combines the practical and the spiritual, which goes along with the belief that the mind influences the body. I've paraphrased Dr. Sun's observations and advice from Honora Lee Wolfe's helpful book *How to Have a Healthy Pregnancy, Healthy Birth with Traditional Chinese Medicine* from Blue Poppy Press. (Note: Sun's months are based on a lunar calendar.)

First Month:
"Embryonic Beginnings"

There will be a preference for delicacies and foods that are sour and delicious. You can eat wheat, but no strong-smelling acrid foods. You should not engage in vigorous activity, sleep should be restful and quiet, and fear should be avoided. An excess of cold will cause pain, while an excess of heat will cause sudden fright, severe abdominal pain, abdominal fullness, and urinary urgency.

Second Month:
"Beginning to Gel"

In this month, the fetus's essence takes shape inside the uterine lining. Avoid spicy and rancid foods. Live in a quiet residence, undisturbed by males. Protect yourself against fright. The yin and yang begin to occupy the channels, and if there is an excess of cold, there will be a miscarriage. If there is too much heat, the fetus will wither.

Third Month:
"Fetal Beginnings"

If you want a male child, hold a bow and arrow. To have a female child, handle pearls. For a beautiful and good child, repeatedly touch a jade seal. If you desire a virtuous and good child, sit formally (still and straight) with a clear and empty mind.

Fourth Month

In this month, the fetus receives the water essence (one of five essences existing in each person), and blood vessels develop. Eat rice and fish broth. The body's six organs develop. You should calm your body, harmonize your mind and ambition, and regulate your diet.

Fifth Month

The fetus receives the fire essence, and this becomes *qi*, the body's life force. During this month, arise early and bathe. Wear clean clothing and have a clean residence. In the morning, inhale the heavenly brightness and avoid contracting colds. Eat rice and wheat, turnips, beef, and mutton. During this month, the fetus's extremities develop, so do not become excessively hungry or overeat.

Avoid dry foods, do not be exposed to baking heat, and do not become excessively fatigued.

Sixth Month

In this month, the metal essence is received, and the fetus develops the sinews and other connective tissue. The body should have some slight exertion; a quiet house is not so necessary. You should eat muscular fowl and the flesh of fierce beasts. You should be out in the fields watching running animals and horses. During this month, the mouth and eyes develop, so the four tastes should be regulated, food should be sweet and delicious, and you should not overeat.

Seventh Month

The fetus receives the water essence, which becomes the bones. You should continue to exert yourself and move your limbs. Live in a dry residence, and avoid cold food and drink, eat rice, and keep your pores closed. During this month, the fetus's skin and hair develop. Do not yell a great deal or cry out, do not wear light clothes, and do not bathe in cold fluids.

Eighth Month

This month, the fetus receives the earth essence and forms the skin. The mind should be peaceful and rested, not causing extremes in the movement of *qi*. During this time, the nine orifices are formed. Do not eat dry foods, and do not inadvertently miss meals.

Ninth Month

In this month, the fetus receives the stone essence, which becomes the skin and hair. All development is complete. Drink sweet wine, eat sweet food, and keep your belt loose. During this month, all the fetus's vessels become continuous. Do not dwell in excessively warm or chilled places.

Tenth Month

The five organs are complete, and the six bowels are connected. The *qi* of heaven and earth has been absorbed into the cinnabar field. Everything is unified, and the personal spirit is complete. Only delivery remains.

Foods That Heal

Much of Dr. Sun's advice is food related. So is my mother's. For Asians, food is used not just for nourishment and enjoyment, but to heal and soothe and balance the body's natural chemistry. A body in balance is a body healthy enough to withstand disease. My parents, for example, blamed my teenage acne on an excess of chocolate. This is a common belief here. However, they attributed the effect on my skin to the "heaty" characteristic of chocolate, which obviously was creating an imbalance in my body.

Even after hearing my mother speak of hot and cold foods for thirty years, I have yet to be able to explain which foods are labeled hot and which are labeled cold—and why. The labels defy Western ideas of hot and cold temperatures; instead, foods are designated hot or cool depending on how they make your body react. For example, tea, whether hot or cold in temperature, is cool. (Perhaps this is why, even on the hottest days, tea drinkers claim that a hot cup of tea cools them down.) Coffee, however, is hot, as are eggs, milk, salty foods, and bitter foods. Fatty foods, be they animal or vegetable, are hot. Juicy fruits and vegetables, slimy foods such as okra, and sour foods are cool.

In Malaysia, pregnant women are told to avoid eating too many cool and wind (which I can only loosely translate as gas-producing) foods. My mother's list of no-nos include: regular and Chinese tea, cucumbers, leafy vegetables, uncooked vegetables, melons, and Chinese cabbage. *Pow sum,* an herb in the ginseng family, can be eaten before labor and delivery to restore balance to the hot/cool system in the body. After labor and delivery, when the body is in a naturally cool state, women eat only hot foods, to restore the body's balance.

One explanation for eating warm foods comes from Wolfe's book. The diet of a pregnant woman, she writes, must be designed to promote blood production for her and the baby. This means eating foods that support the spleen, the organ the Chinese believe creates *qi* and blood from the purest part of what we eat. Foods must be warmed to body temperature before the spleen can do its work.

Chilled and raw foods require the spleen to work harder and leave less energy for making *qi* and blood.

My aunt also warns against upsetting the yin and yang balance in the body. Some foods are labeled yin foods; others are yang. For example, you shouldn't eat too much melon—a yin food—without balancing it with, say, a bucket of fried chicken—a yang food.

Cravings

Cravings are one of the best parts of pregnancy. When else in our lives do we have license to eat anything and everything because of a craving? The Chinese agree wholeheartedly. Yet, when a craving arises, it should be satisfied with a *very small amount* of that food, even if you do not ordinarily eat the food or consider it healthy. Asian medical texts encourage the mother to satisfy the craving even if the food is revolting or strange! If a small amount does not suffice, the craving is probably inappropriate. So don't pig out on whatever it is you are craving—you'll probably regret it later. In fact, the Japanese do not believe in cravings at all. A mother should have more discipline than that!

Exercise

Exercise is an important part of pregnancy, relieving the annoying aches and pains that go with carrying an extra twenty to thirty pounds, helping tone the body for the stress of labor and delivery, and promoting a sense of control and well-being in the mother. That's the Western explanation. The Chinese one goes something like this: Exercise improves the function of the spleen, the organ that produces the important *qi* and blood. It also helps the health of the liver, which controls the flow of *qi* throughout the body. (A stagnant liver plays a part in morning sickness and may cause a difficult labor.) Exercise also releases the excess heat caused by internal stress on the body, strengthens the heart and lungs, and helps relieve constipation. Finally, exercise helps guard against the accumulation of "dampness" in the body, which otherwise might turn into fat. Sounds like a good reason to me!

Home Remedies

These remedies are collected from mothers and grandmas around the world. I take no responsibility for their effectiveness, but perhaps one or two are worth a try!

Backaches

Japanese women take baths in the volcanic hot springs called *o-nsen* to relieve backaches. Or they heat a stone or brick, wrap it in a towel, and place it on their backs, much like a heating pad. If you don't live near a volcano or want to burn one of your towels, try a hot shower or a massage. My mother suggested using *hong ewe,* hundred-herb oil, for a massage. If that's not available, use any oil—and any masseuse—that feels good, but keep in mind, massaging with *hong ewe* will also help prevent stretch marks! (Check your local Asian market store for *hong ewe*.)

Colds

Grate some ginger into a cup of green tea topped with green onion. No sugar allowed, but you can use soy sauce to taste.

Constipation

In Japan, they make a tea with an herb called *doku dami*, which is dried in the dark and then ground. It's also supposed to keep you looking young.

Eat oranges or oats to relieve constipation.

Eggplant is known to cause diarrhea in pregnant woman, so it may help constipation, but eat it sparingly.

Cramps

Cramps, some say, are a result of too many yin foods. Balance with yang foods.

Eat pears and watermelon.

Flatulence

Ginger, boiled or sweetened, helps relieve gas.

Headaches

A Japanese grandma suggests that mothers should drink a cup of *ma-cha*, the green tea used for the Japanese tea ceremony, sweetened with honey and lemon, to relieve headaches.

Morning Sickness:
Ginger Tea

My cousin Pey Pey and my friend Young drank enough ginger tea to support the whole ginger industry. To make the tea, Young boiled four ounces of ginger in hot water and sweetened it with honey or sugar. Pey Pey made individual cups of hot water with a few slices of ginger. Either way, both made it through their first trimester with few complaints.

Nasal Congestion

Try this at home: Make a Japanese *ship-pu* to wrap around your neck. Mix pan-fried green onion with flour to make a paste. Then smear the paste on a piece of gauze and wrap it around your neck.

✧ ✧ ✧

With herbal remedies and the like, I am first American and then Chinese. Often, it surprises me to hear just how many people believe in the small jars of oils and powders that stocked my parents' medicine chest. It isn't surprising, really. Chinese medicine and all its offshoots have been practiced for over two thousand years. There are more Chinese—and more Asians in general—than any other nationality on earth. Surely there must be something valid about the practices of so many people.

These days, the special herbs and ointments of my childhood have a different effect. When I smell the licorice smell of *hong ewe* or feel the sting of *ipoh ewe,* more than anything I am transported to the comforts of home. It almost doesn't matter if they work: I am made happy by the flood of memories, the remembrances of being cared for. As I take the oily bottle of *ipoh ewe* out of the closet to soothe my son's insect bites, I am trapped between my two worlds, feeling now more Chinese than American. Perhaps one day he will remember the smell, and with it, remember my love, too.

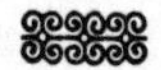

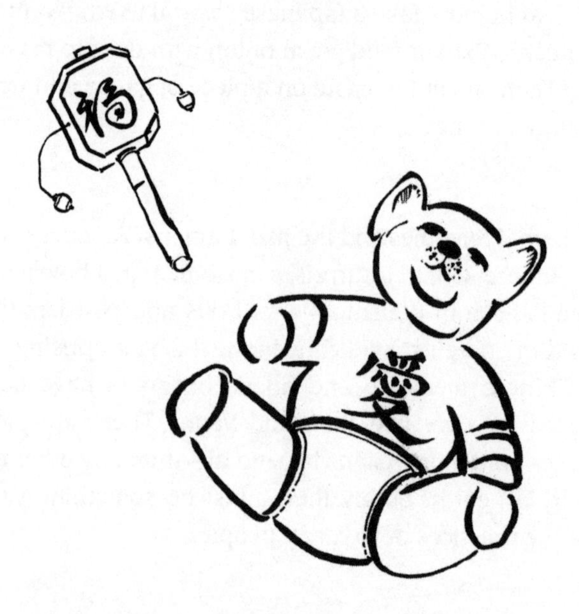

4

Boy or Girl? The Secrets of the Five-Yen Coin

Roving
in the trees,

a golden pear
appeared on a stem
before my eyes.

I smiled slowly,
trying to grasp it
in my hand . . .

but it was made of pure light
floating through my body.

I bore
a gentle girl.

KOREAN BIRTH DREAM

FORETELLING THE SEX OF THE COMING BABY is an endless source of amusement for parents, family, friends, and sometimes even strangers on the street. I think I've heard them all: your stomach is flat, you must be having a girl. Your stomach is pointy, you must be having a boy. Your face is soft, it's a girl. The baby is kicking? Must be a boy. The variations are endless. At my baby shower, a woman who had recently arrived from China told me that if the mother's face is gentle, it will be a girl. If it is tired and drawn, it is a boy.

"What will I have?" I asked.

She was caught. With a nervous laugh, she said I looked very pretty. What else could she say? She was a guest in my house! It must be a girl, she said, nodding.

I had a boy.

In Asia, of course, sons were—and in some places still are—considered paramount. As one older Korean put it, "Daughters result in two sorrows—one when they're born and one when they're married." The traditional *Book of Odes* describes Chinese parents' similar attitude:

A son is born.
He is placed upon a bed,
and clothed with brilliant stuffs.

A daughter is born.
They place her on the ground;
they wrap her in common cloths.

Yet apart from their place in the family hierarchy, girls were beloved for their own sakes. There is a tale from the Sung Dynasty in China about a father who loved his daughter so much, he taught her every conceivable branch of learning. In the end, he was so enamored of her character, he couldn't find a man suitable to marry her.

Manu, the revered Chinese philosopher, has this to say about girls: "A householder must consider his wife and son as his own body; his daughter, as the highest object of tenderness."

In Japan and China, it was often preferable that a girl is born first, a girl who would be trained as a mother's helper. The ideal family, says one Japanese-American, would be a girl, followed by two sons—two, in case one son passed away.

How to Make a Boy or a Girl

With boys so prized in Asia, the old wives' tales about how to conceive a boy or a girl are polished to a high degree. Even here in America, there are many theories. Manu wrote, thousands of years ago, that "on the even nights are conceived sons; on the odd nights daughters; therefore, let the man who wishes for a son, approach his wife in due season on the even nights; but a boy is in truth produced by the greater quality of the male strength; and a girl by the greater quality of the female."

If it is true that the male's sexual performance can determine the sex of the child, how much more suspect is the Japanese belief that the dominant partner in the marriage has his or her say? As the myth goes, if the wife is the dominant member of the household, the baby will be a boy. If the husband rules, the child will be a girl. And traditionally, Korean women were told they must not giggle at their wedding. Laughing or smiling would produce girls.

Even your home's *feng shui,* the Taoist concept of balance in the environment, can affect the sex of your child. One man in old Beijing who had four daughters asked a geomancer to come to his home to uncover the problem. The practitioner said the chimney of the missionary across the street was interfering with his *feng shui*. The man approached the missionary, who dismantled the chimney. Success! He and his wife had two fine sons.

If you want a boy or a girl baby, traditional Chinese medicine has some key strategies to try. Practitioners believe that male-producing sperm is quicker but short-lived, while female-producing sperm is slower but lives longer. For intercourse after ovulation: If you want a boy, make sure the male partner is not fully inserted when he ejaculates. This allows the faster male sperm to reach the descending egg before the slower female sperm. Deep insertion after ovulation will place a greater number of female sperm closer to the egg. For intercourse before ovulation, the situation is reversed. Shallow intercourse makes a female baby more likely, since the longer-living female sperm are more likely to survive to meet the egg. Deeper intercourse increases the percentage of male sperm likely to reach the egg.

Foods can also determine the sex of the baby. For a boy, the Japanese believe that the father should eat lots of vegetables, the mother lots of meat. Boys can also be created by eating root vegetables such as turnips and carrots—the association of the long "root" is obvious. For girls, the fare is reversed; the father should eat lots of meat, and the mother should eat lots of vegetables.

If you're convinced that you're having a boy when you wanted a girl, or vice versa, don't worry: One Korean doctor believes the sex of a child is not fixed until a few weeks after conception. He prescribes a medicine that can help change the sex of the unborn child. Based on the theory that foods have either yang (male) properties and some have yin (female) properties, his remedy involves the mother's swallowing a boiled herbal concoction. If she wants a boy, the medicine is made from yang herbs; to produce a girl, it is made from yin herbs.

Is It a Boy or Girl? Telltale Signs

Myths abound about ways to tell if you're having a boy or a girl. Many transcend cultures—wide hips and a heavy bottom foretell a girl (or too much ice cream) in both

China and the United States. Most likely, you'll show some telltale signs. If you're a bettor, you can weigh the odds. Or, as we do here in America, have an ultrasound before you buy the three-pack of pink onesies. Here are some common clues:

- If you're carrying the baby low, it is a boy. If you're carrying high, it is a girl (Taiwan).
- If you crave fruits, it is a boy. If you desire flowers, it is a girl (Philippines).
- If your right side bulges, it is a boy. If your left side bulges, it is a girl (Philippines).
- If your face is stern, it is a boy. If your face is soft and gentle, it is a girl (Malaysia, China).
- If you have an active, kicking baby, it is almost universally pegged to be a boy.
- If you have a strong pulse in your left wrist, it is a boy. A strong pulse in your right wrist indicates a girl. If the pulse is stronger nearer the wrist, it is a boy. A stronger pulse nearer to your elbow means you will have a girl (China).

If these are too vague for you, try the Japanese five-yen coin test. Pluck a piece of your hair from your head and tie a five-yen coin to it. (If you don't have access to a five-yen coin, try a subway token, or any coin with a hole.) Hold the dangling coin over the back of your hand. If it spins in a circle, it is a girl. If it swings back and forth, it is a boy.

Dreaming of Babies

Analyzing your birth dreams may also be helpful. In a study of over two thousand birth dreams in Korea, Fred Jeremy Seligson came up with these baby symbols and the sex they represent:

Boys	suns, persimmons, red peppers, carps, dragons, snakes, tigers, horses, and pigs
Girls	flowers, apples, butterflies, cherries, strawberries, shellfish, owls, rabbits, jewels, and hens

A further analysis, says Seligson, would take into consideration the yin/yang aspects of the dream. For example, the colors you see in the dream are less important than their shade: a brilliant color such as a diamond or a sun is yang (male). A shadowy hue, such as a cloud, an object indoors or in a cave, would be yin (female). Something sweet or cool, such as an apple or green vegetable, is female. A sour, hot item, such as a red pepper or a tart fruit, is male.

Not surprisingly, the connections are often Freudian. For example, objects that move upward with force, such as a powerful dragon flying into the sky, are male. Objects that slide down or are passive, such as waterfalls or raindrops, are female. Items seen on the tops of mountains foretell boys; items seen on precipices such as cliffs mean girls. Numbers of objects also have meaning. A solitary object, like one pepper, refers to males. Three objects also refer to males—three meaning the penis and two testicles. Half objects (half moons) or objects split in two (butterflies) foretell girls, who open to receive life.

The many tests, symbols, and clues used to foretell the sex of your baby can be fun. But if these symbols only serve to frustrate your best guess, just remember that the game only lasts nine months. And for those of you who just can't wait, there's always ultrasound. As your pregnancy comes to a close, the uppermost concern in your mind will not be whether you have enough mint-green pajamas. As the weeks go by and delivery day comes closer, your thoughts will turn more toward seeing and holding that precious child, no matter what sex it is.

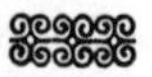

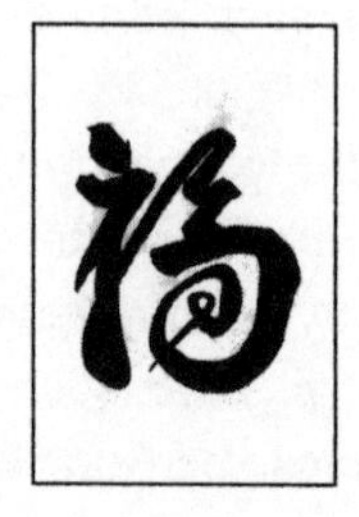

5

The Lucky Day of Birth

My little baby, little boy blue,
is as sweet as sugar and cinnamon, too;
isn't this precious darling of ours
sweeter than dates and cinnamon flowers?
CHINESE NURSERY RHYME

IT BEGINS WITH A HARD CRAMP, perhaps a whoosh of water, perhaps a vague feeling that something about your body has changed. The moment has arrived! If you lived in old Asia, you might begin labor already confined to your bedroom, a small extra room, or, if you were wealthy, a separate house built for the occasion. Women in labor were considered "unclean," and were kept away from the rest of the household. In Japan, women retired to their rooms twenty-one days before the expected delivery. In India, the woman was kept in a small room with windows and doors tightly closed. The worst beds, the oldest bedding were used for her birth chamber. She was so isolated that sometimes the only midwife who would help her was of a lower caste. The midwife knew little, if anything, about hygiene—a far cry from today's supersterilized hospital rooms. In Japan, such women were called *samba-san,* "women in reduced circumstances," and had no training except from other *samba-san.*

In China, the day of your child's birth might start with a prayer to the goddess who helped you conceive, an offering of sweetmeats, the burning of incense. A strong herbal potion was mixed and swallowed to ease the strains of labor. In the Philippines, the house was prepared. All the doors and windows were flung wide open—a gesture symbolic of the child's easy passage. A knot of fresh ginger was crushed in the doorway by a menstruating woman, a wish for less painful contractions.

Want an Easy Labor?

Not surprisingly, the dangers and pain of labor have created many a myth and many a potential—or hoped-for—remedy. In China, a bride entering the home of her husband for the first time is carried over a pan of burning coals. The pan is put in place by two women whose husbands and children are living. Thus, it is said, the bride will pass successfully through labor.

In the ancient Kingdom of Sukothai, now Thailand, fourteenth-century mothers used clay figures of women to transfer the dangers of childbirth onto inanimate objects. To perform this magical transfer, women decapitated these feminine effigies just before the onset of labor. Only then would they be safe from the perils of childbirth.

In the Philippines, a woman could avoid a difficult labor if she took the following steps. She should:

wear a belt made from monkey or snakeskin
step over abaca fiber
open the doors and windows just before delivery
rub her stomach with the roasted feces of earthworms

She would have a hard time bearing a child if she:

attended a funeral
walked over a string or any striped object
lay on the floor against the grain
moved into a new house

They Call It Labor in Asia, Too

When the hard work began, Asian women traditionally labored in silence. To cry out or moan was a sign of weakness, a loss of that important Asian commodity called face in English. The Chinese say, "A Chinese woman who approaches childbirth with fear of the birth pains is considered a coward not worthy of life. Birth is a woman's career."

In Japan, women who gave in to the pain and screamed were said to become poor mothers. Filipina mothers believed it was a sign of difficult labors to come.

The enduring myth—who knows where it started—

about Asian women is that they're so strong, so stoic, that they give birth squatting in a field. In the West, we are just beginning to experiment once again with different birthing positions. I believe it was Louis XIV who made laboring lying flat on your back fashionable. (It is said that this position gave him the best view of the birth of his children.) Through the years, this position of labor became viewed as correct and the squatting or standing positions were seen as primitive. Research now shows that these alternative laboring positions can help shorten labor—gravity helps!—and relieve some of the discomfort.

It seems that Asian women knew all this long ago. A book on labor written in the 1800s has a chapter entitled "Characteristic Labor Scenes Among the Yellow, Black, and Red Races." In it, the author, a Western doctor, describes the typical Japanese birth. In the Tokugawa period, a birthing framework was devised that looked like a big chair with no legs. Over the years, this framework was downscaled to a pile of futons piled to support the back and provide a place to kneel. The baby is delivered as the woman supports herself on her knees and toes, bending forward and grasping a sturdy low table or her midwife, who assists by rubbing her abdomen. Sometimes another midwife stands behind her to rub her head or lend support, even hugging her abdomen to exert some pressure. After birth, the woman will sit up on this futon bed for three days. Only on the fourth day may she finally lie down.

In the past, Asian women had a number of other methods to move labor along, most of which sound more painful to me than labor itself. One Japanese-American woman says that when her mother was long past her due date, her father tied an *obi* (wide sash) tightly around her abdomen. She was then suspended upside down until she went into labor.

Long ago, women in Thailand were given a hand by two women who seated themselves, one on each side of her. While the laboring woman lay on her back, these women would push and pull the abdomen forward and backward for three to five hours. If labor became difficult, one attendant would stand up and stomp on the mother's upper abdomen, taking care not to tread on the baby. If things were really difficult, the woman was hung from bands wrapped around her arms and secured to the ceiling. One of the attendants would then wrap her arms around the laboring woman, above the fetus, and hang from this poor woman until the child was born.

In Burma, childbirth sounded like a game of mud wrestling. According to one book on labor, the laboring woman was forced to run about the room naked, while half a dozen women squeezed her abdomen and beat it with pillows. When the woman collapsed with exhaustion—not surprising—the other women used their hands to press out the child. In some cases, the mother lay on her back while the midwife sat on her and pressed the child out with her feet. I wonder if they offered an epidural for this one?

Chinese women traditionally labored in an armchair or a bed. If the baby was delayed, they once again called upon the gods for help. Help could take many forms, as this excerpt from *Rituals for Birth* describes:

> My labor went on and on; through that night, through sunset of the next day. In the dim, hazy world I lived in, I knew people were gathering outside my bed. A Taoist priest came and muttered prayers in my ear. I wanted to shout to him, "Speak to the one down there; the one who refuses to come out! Don't prattle to me!" He only waved some charms written on yellow paper, burned one, and mixed it with water. This I had to drink, to make the child come.
>
> It did not. More hours had gone by when I heard the sounds of people in the room. Li drew open the bed curtains and told me to look at the doorway. There were the puppeteers with their gay, bright puppets. For the first time in many hours, my heart lifted. One of the puppets was an image of Mother [goddess of childbirth], while the others were her helpers. They danced and turned in the doorway, and it almost seemed the goddess was there. Then, since I was old for a first birth and my labor was long, the puppeteer came and put the image of Mother on my stomach. Three times the tiny goddess moved swiftly down to the birth-opening. So the child should move, as quickly and as easily.

Born Under Lucky Stars: The Birth

The moment the child arrives is like none other. To finally see its precious face, its tiny hands, to hold its body against yours . . . it is a moment you will never forget. And, if you believe the myths, neither will your child.

The hour, day, month, and year a child is born—the Chinese call them the Eight Characters, the Koreans the Four Pillars—are considered so significant that the child's entire life will be ruled by them. Like a person's astrological sign, these heavenly dates can foretell if a child will be successful, wealthy, and blessed with good fortune or if his or her life will be short and full of sadness. Upon a child's birth, fortune-tellers and soothsayers are hired to read the future of this new life. Each hour of each day, each day of each month carries certain divine predictions. For example, in the Ming dynasty novel *The Golden Lotus,* one immortal uses the Eight Characters to divine the future of Hsi-men Ch'ing. He is born between the seventh and eighth month, which gives him physical vigor. The day of his birth foretells that he will profit from his abilities, the hour that he will have a career of great dignity. He is born in the year of the Tiger, which makes him passionate and decisive.

The Eight Characters continue to be important throughout a person's life. For example, when a potential spouse is found, the Eight Characters are consulted again to see if the two will be a good match. A sheet of paper on which the characters are written is placed on the family shrine. If nothing bad happens in three days—no plates are broken, no one becomes ill—then the couple is blessed.

A fortune-teller might also divine the child's future health and prospects. The Chinese believe that each person has some of the five elements in his or her constitution: metal, wood, water, fire, and earth. If metal, wood, or earth is lacking—how they tell this I don't know—that element's character is incorporated into that child's name. If water or fire is absent, that is considered a good omen. A child with too much fire could be injured by fire in his life; a child with too much water needs to be watched, for she might drown.

At the moment of birth, Filipinas have another ritual meant to affect the future life of the child. A bamboo box, left open in the delivery room to "catch" the baby's first cry, is quickly shut so that the child will not be a crybaby. Black ashes are rubbed on the baby's palms and feet so he or she will be a good climber.

And don't forget those lucky stars: The Asians believe that the astrological calendar also affects the future personality and temperament of the child. In this country, most Westerners know of the Asian zodiac from news reports around Chinese New Year or from the paper placemat at the local Chinese take-out, but many Asians take it a bit more seriously. The zodiac is based on the moon, which is said to deeply influence the moment of birth.

(The moon is also said to govern the fluids in the body and to represent the soul's passions, desires, and feelings.) Unlike the Western zodiac, which names each month for a different star formation, the Asian zodiac names a cycle of twelve years after twelve animals, each with its own traits and characteristics. Every person born in a particular year will manifest the signs of that particular animal. The child born in the year of the ram, for example, will grow up artistic and compassionate. When my first son was born, one uncle sent me the characteristics of my son's animal, the loyal and trustworthy dog. We shall see if he lives up to his destiny!

What will your child's personality be like? Consult this list to find your child's birth animal, and read on to see the basic traits associated with that year. (If you don't find your year, then count back by increments of twelve to find your birth animal.)

Rat	thrifty, quick-tempered, charming	1960, 1972, 1984, 1996
Ox	stubborn, patient, trusting, dependable	1961, 1973, 1985, 1997
Tiger	sensitive, passionate, and daring	1962, 1974, 1986, 1998
Rabbit	affectionate, cautious, good head for business	1963, 1975, 1987, 1999
Dragon	full of vitality and strength, sets high standards	1964, 1976, 1988, 2000

Snake	deep thinker and soft-spoken	1965, 1977, 1989, 2001
Horse	cheerful, perceptive and quick-witted, loves to be where the action is	1966, 1978, 1990, 2002
Ram	strong beliefs, compassionate, artistic	1967, 1979, 1991, 2003
Monkey	inventor and improviser	1968, 1980, 1992, 2004
Rooster	sharp and neat, extravagant in dress, prefers working alone	1969, 1981, 1993, 2005
Dog	loyal, trustworthy and faithful, makes a good but reluctant leader	1970, 1982, 1994, 2006
Pig	studious, well informed, reliable	1971, 1983, 1995, 2007

The Twelve Animals

There are many stories about the way the twelve animals came to be named as those of the zodiac. One legend tells that Buddha invited all the animals to a banquet on his last day on earth. These twelve animals were the only ones who appeared, and as a token of his gratitude, Buddha named a year after each one, in the order of their arrival.

In another version, my personal favorite, the Jade Emperor invited all the animals to a race in which they had to cross a large river. The first twelve animals across the river, he announced, would become the twelve animals of the zodiac. The contest caused much excitement in the animal world. At the time, the cat and the rat were the best of friends, spending the entire day in each other's company. When the contest was announced, they worried that they might be too small to get to the river quickly.

"The ox wakes up very early," said the cat. "Let's ask him to wake us up early on the day of the race so we may have a chance."

On race day, the ox kindly woke the cat and the rat before the rooster even opened an eye. Since they were sleepy, the ox offered them a ride to the river on his back. As the first light broke, they reached the river, the first to arrive. They were so excited; one of the three would be the first in the zodiac! The selfish rat, however, was still scheming: How could he make sure he was first across and the first animal to begin the zodiac?

He hit upon a plan. When the three animals reached the middle of the river, the rat said to the cat, "Look upon the fine landscape on the far shore!" The cat stood up on tiptoes to see what his friend was pointing at. At that moment, the rat pushed his friend into the water. The ox, looking back to see why his back was lighter, saw the horse and the tiger gaining on him, and so forgot about the cat, and swam on. When the ox reached the shore, the rat jumped out of his ear. Startled, the ox paused, and the rat raced to victory.

He was followed in turn by the ox, the tiger, the rabbit,

the dragon, the horse, the sheep, the monkey, the rooster, and the dog. The last was the lazy pig. The Jade Emperor named each animal in turn. As he came to the end, the soaking wet cat clambered ashore. "What about me?" he cried.

"I'm sorry," said the Emperor. "You are too late."

With that, the cat screamed, "It's that sneaky rat's fault. I am going to eat him up!"

Since then, the rat and the cat have been mortal enemies, and the rat, ashamed of how he won first place, hides in dark corners and comes out only at night.

Birth Announcements: Red Eggs, Pig's Feet, and Strings of Peppers

There are other rituals that announce the arrival of the child to family and friends. Instead of beribboned birth announcements, the new father in China sends gifts of money and wine to his in-laws. Special ribbons placed around the wine jar signify a boy or a girl.

Red eggs are sent to close family and friends who might be giving gifts. The number of eggs you receive depends on whether the new baby is a boy or girl: even numbers for a girl, odd for a boy.

A wealthy family in Canton might also send out bowls of pig's feet cooked with ginger, sugar, and soy sauce. In some other areas of China, parents send out boxes of fruits to announce the arrival of the child. Return gifts might include two kinds of cake, brown sugar, millet, eggs, and walnut meats—foods that the mother is allowed to eat during the first three days after the birth.

In Korea, strings of red peppers are hung outside the door to announce the arrival of a boy; straw and charcoal are hung if it's a girl. These festive garlands also keep away visitors for the required twenty-one days before mother and baby can be viewed by non-family members.

For most, little else is done on that momentous day. Mother and baby are encouraged to rest. Visitors, especially non-family members, are kept away for days, even weeks, probably to protect the mother and child from germs. Perhaps because of high infant mortality in ancient times, the Japanese traditionally wait seven days before even naming the child. In China, the maternal grandmother waits three days before visiting her daughter with gifts for the child.

The Afterbirth

Little attention is paid to what happens to the placenta and umbilical cord here in the West. After our son was born, my husband cut the cord that bound my life to our son's. I have no idea what happened to it. In Asia, however, the placenta and umbilical cord are treated with great reverence and respect, myths about them sometimes taking on a life of their own.

In most Asian cultures, the placenta is buried under the house, or in the earth around the house. There are differing reasons and beliefs surrounding this. Some do it to ward off evil spirits. Others believe the placenta somehow forms a mystical link between the child and the home that will, later in life, draw the child back to his or her birthplace. For some cultures, the placenta represents good fortune. Once it is buried, those who step near the placenta burial spot will be graced with fertility.

Great care is taken with the placenta; it is not just dropped into a hole in the ground. The Japanese, for example, place the placenta in an earthen jar. If the child is a boy, a stick of India ink and a writing brush will be placed with it and buried within the family gate so that he will remain in the family. A girl's placenta is buried outside the family gate because she will, upon marriage, become part of another family.

The placenta was once regarded as so important in Korea that the nobility and royalty reserved special spots for placental burials in royal cemeteries. The placenta was placed in a small jar, which was fit into a larger jar—perhaps symbolic of its origins.

As for the umbilical cord, the Filipinas believed if you kept it in the ceiling, your child would grow strong. Tied to a tree, it would prevent stomachaches. Most of all, it was important to keep it intact so future children would not quarrel. In 1800s Japan, the umbilical cord was wrapped in several sheets of white paper, and then in a special paper on which the mother's and father's full names were written. If the child died, the cord was buried with him. If he lived to adulthood, he carried the cord along with him until he died, and it was buried with him.

Very few of these birthing rituals have made it to our shores. Most Asian-Americans give birth in a hospital, not in a separate room at home. Once the child is born, perhaps a fortune-teller may be called by an older grandmother, or a relative may note the child's birth year. Certainly no one I know carries her umbilical cord with her!

What does remain, however, is the awesome respect for life that is reflected in these rituals. The silence of the laboring woman could be seen as the mightiest of strengths, the confidence that a woman was formed to give birth—something that we have lost a little in our antiseptic world of doctors, epidurals, and monitors. The horoscope taken at the instance of birth is an acknowledgment that this child matters, that this new human being has created a ripple in the vast ocean of the universe. The respect for the placenta, for the umbilical cord that nourished, protected, and sustained this new life, shows also the great value placed on the life itself. We may read about these rituals, these myths, with a sense of foreignness, even of embarrassment. But remember, too, the truths and beauty of new life that these rituals enshrine. Most of these rituals were practiced long ago, but the truths—the strength of women, the connection to the world around us, the respect of life—are part of us and, I hope, will continue to live throughout the generations to come.

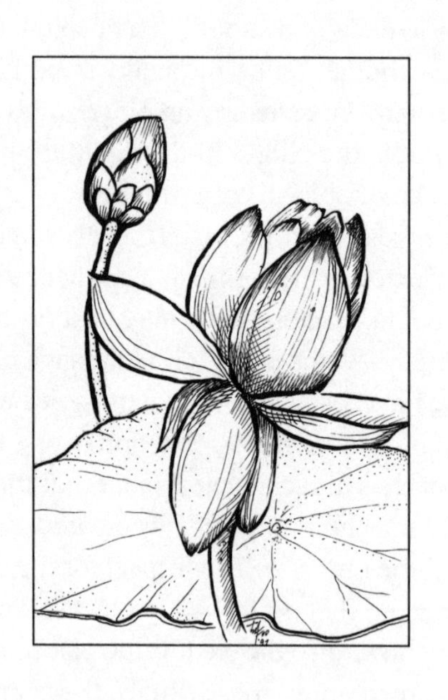

6

The New Mother: Traditions, Tales, and Recipes to Soothe, Comfort, and Heal

She bathes
in a clear stream,
secluded by scented
trees, under glowing sun.

While in paradise,
a tiger enters her womb,
and she sets a moonstone
on her finger.

A star falls
on her breast.

She snips lilies
into the folds
of her dress

going home
with her child.

KOREAN BIRTH DREAM

When my son was born, I stayed in the hospital for three days, one day longer than the insurance company normally would allow, because of complications. When my mother gave birth to my brother in 1971, she stayed in her New York hospital for a week. When my grandmother gave birth to my mother in prewar Malaysia, she followed the old ways and stayed in her bed, confined to her room, for one whole month.

"Sitting the month," as it is called in Chinese, is an intense healing time for the new mother. Freed from her normal household and family responsibilities, she is allowed only to sit in bed and look after her new infant. (In very strict households, even the husband traditionally was not allowed to enter and disturb her!) The practice continues today in many Asian countries. In Korea and Japan, the mother rests in her room for twenty-one days. For the first three days, the Japanese mother is kept sitting on her futon night and day. Only after three days is she allowed to lie down. In Thailand, the mother is confined for thirty days for the first child, five fewer days for each successive baby. Sitting the month is such an accepted ritual that one mother in China exclaimed, "I had no idea it was a cultural practice. I thought it was science!"

There are other, more quirky, aspects to the traditional confinement. In many countries, women are not allowed to bathe or wash their hair for one month after giving birth, or they'll suffer from headaches and arthritis for the rest of their life. In Malaysia, the mother can be sponged with water boiled with special herbs or lemongrass to help remove wind, as my aunt explains. The water used to sponge the mother can be cool—Malaysia has a tropical climate—but it needs to have been boiled and then cooled.

Koreans also believe that a woman should not bathe for five to seven days after birth or she'll develop muscle aches, especially when it rains.

Great care is taken to keep mother and child very warm, even on the hottest days of summer. A postpartum woman is considered "cool" and needs the heat to bring about full health. (Interestingly, I once saw a Western medical study that showed that heat promotes healing, especially after blood loss.) In Korea and Japan, the mother is dressed in long underwear, the heat is turned up, and mother and child are bundled together with heavy quilts. Older Koreans love to tell stories of the arthritis they developed because one patch of skin was showing outside the quilt!

To heal the womb during this time, the Malaysians and the Thai use heat. In Malaysia, a *tunku* (a heavy round iron with a handle) or a stone is heated over a charcoal fire, wrapped in cloth, and pushed against the abdomen. Special leaves are also heated and placed on the abdomen. In ancient Thailand, they took this practice to the extreme: The mother was placed on a bamboo cot under which sat a pot of burning coals to "dry the womb." When it became too hot, the mother was flipped, much like a grilled fish. The heat was sometimes so great that the mother would blister all over her body. Still the treatment would continue for two or three weeks. Thank goodness, a hot water bottle placed on the belly is all that remains of this custom today!

In the Philippines, special women vigorously massage the new mother to push her organs back in place— "a must in the villages," says my Filipina friend. Called *hilot,* these women use pressure points and holds that rival a great wrestler's to work you over. This massage is performed at least three times in the first two months postpartum.

Instead of warm sitz baths to heal the perineum after labor, Filipina villagers used to sit over a pot full of steaming guava leaves as many times as possible.

When I had my first child, my mother was adamant that I spend as much time as possible sitting and resting. Even a gentle stroll around the neighborhood was frowned upon. Many Asian-Americans I've spoken to have described "sitting for a month," leading me to believe that though this custom might not be practiced, its influence is felt here, too. Oddly enough, the many superstitions and rituals that go along with this time period are also heeded by many—though most would not admit to it. One Chinese-American professor says her mother warned her about the cold, but she didn't listen. And she now wishes she had.

"Two weeks after the baby was born, I used cold water to wash a diaper," she says. "My mother told me not to, but I told her I really couldn't see any harm to it. A few days later, I developed a swollen joint in my hand that still hurts today. With the next child, born in July, I went out to take a walk. My mother told me to put on a hat; the wind was cold. Really, I told her, it is the middle of July. You know, I developed the weirdest headache that day. It was so strange that I didn't go out for another month. It hasn't come back since, but it made a believer out of me."

Food and Recipes to Heal and Soothe

For many Asians, foods and herbs form the basis of healing. Koreans, for example, use herbal medicines, squash cooked with honey or in soup, and meat soup made from bones to restore new mothers' strength. In Malaysia, special "heaty" foods are prescribed by knowing mothers and old aunties. My mother discouraged drinks of cool water or liquids, even in late August. Tea made by pouring boiling water over fried rice—not the house special, just raw rice that was toasted—and ginger was the drink of choice. (It's supposed to relieve flatulence.) In Malaysia, my aunties prescribe special herbs for boiling with drinks or making chicken soup; *pow sum* gives heat to the body and is eaten on the twelfth day after birth, and *tong kuei* is taken for strength.

Kidney, pig's maw, liver, pepper, and fish such as pomfret are also said to produce heat, as well as providing the nutrition the mother needs. Fruits and vegetables, especially those belonging to the melon family, are too cool for this period of time. Foods cooked in ginger and sesame oil are popular. The following are some recipes I've collected.

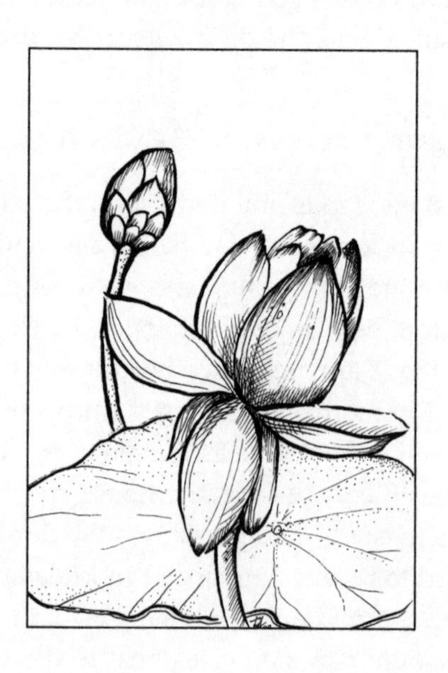

DRUNKEN CHICKEN

(reprinted by permission of Martin Yan)

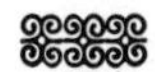

You might notice that all the ingredients are "heaty." Wood ear, available at Asian grocery stores, is a type of fungus also called cloud's ear. Interestingly enough, Yan mentions that a group of researchers at the University of Minnesota recently found that wood ear inhibits blood clots.

Wine Sauce:
2½ cups rice wine
1½ cups sherry wine
1½ teaspoons salt
1½ teaspoons sugar

Other Ingredients:
2¼ pounds whole chicken
2 tablespoons oil
2 green onions, cut into ½-inch strips
1 cup raw peanuts
½ cup sliced ginger
6 ounces lean pork, cut into 1½-inch chunks
1 ounce wood ear, soaked and sliced

1. Combine ingredients for wine sauce in a small bowl. Put aside.

2. Cut meat from whole chicken into 2-inch cubes. Heat oil in wok over high heat; add green onion, peanuts, and ginger, stirring for 1 minute. Add chicken and pork, stirring for 1½–2 minutes.
3. Mix in wood ear and wine sauce. Bring to a boil. Reduce heat to low, cover, and simmer for 17–20 minutes.
4. Serve warm or cold.

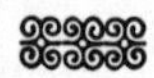

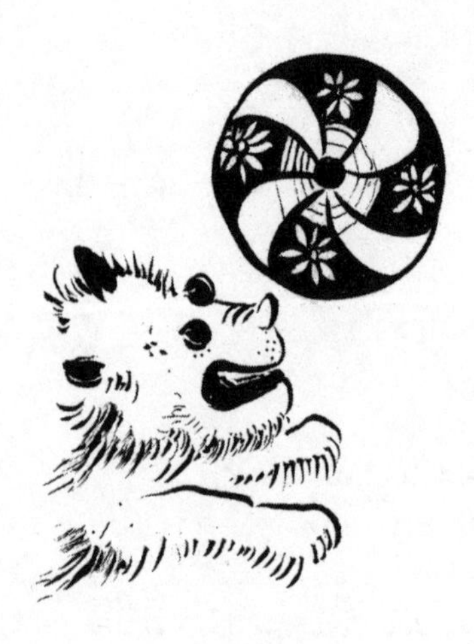

AUNTY'S KIDNEY AND LIVER STEW

My cousin loves this dish, which is perfect for "sitting the month." There are no quantities to the ingredients; like most home chefs, my aunt cooks "to taste."

kidney, washed thoroughly, sliced and scored
liver, washed thoroughly, sliced and scored
soy sauce
pepper
sesame oil
ginger, sliced into thin strips
rice wine
pinch of sugar (optional)

1. Marinate the kidney and liver in soy sauce, pepper, and sesame oil.
2. Fry the ginger in a little oil and add the seasoned kidney and liver. Do not overcook.
3. Add the rice wine to make it soupy. If the wine is not sweet enough, add a pinch of sugar. Serve.

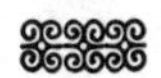

MOM'S HERBED CHICKEN ESSENCE

My mom serves this soup whenever someone's sick. The purest chicken soup, it's great for restoring strength.

1 small, skinless chicken with wing tips chopped off
8–10 slices of *pow sum* or ginger

1. In the top half of a double boiler, balance the chicken on top of a small, upturned bowl.
2. Add ¼ cup water and the slices of *pow sum* or ginger. (Available in Chinese grocery stores, *pow sum* restores a woman's strength and should only be eaten after the twelfth day postpartum.)
3. Boil for three hours over low heat. Spice as desired and serve. (Mom adds soy sauce and salt, or throws in vegetables and cut-up chicken.)

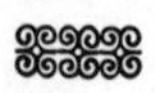

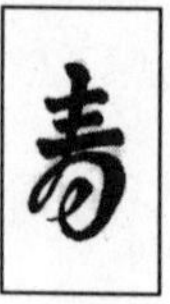

YOUNG MCGRADY'S SEAWEED SOUP

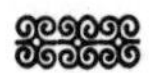

For the Koreans, even among the Korean-Americans, seaweed soup is the soup du jour for the first weeks postpartum. Many mothers drink this soup three to *seven* times a day! One Korean-American woman tells me the soup is full of iron, good for "purifying the blood," she says. She also admits to having disliked the taste until the birth of her fourth child.

My Korean-American friend Young loves this soup, which has been served at every birthday she can remember. "I guess the first time I had it was in the womb!" she says. Now that she's pregnant, she drinks it several times a week. Even her Western husband loves it. Each family has its own variations, but here's Young's, which is less seasoned than most to preserve the essence of the seaweed:

1 lb. beef, any cut you use to make soup
water in 10-qt. pot
dried seaweed, rinsed to remove any sand and softened
in water for 5 minutes
salt
soy sauce

1. Boil beef in water for about 2 hours until the meat is tender and the broth is savory.
2. Remove the bones. Cut the meat into bite-size pieces, and put it back in the pot.
3. Add the seaweed, chopped into quarters.
4. Simmer for another hour. Season to taste and serve.

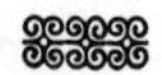

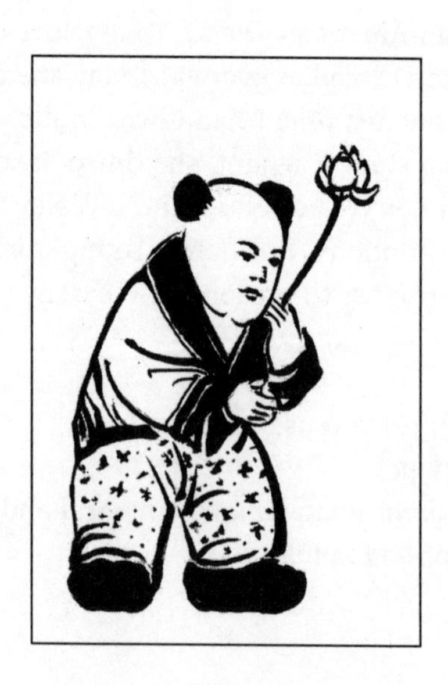

Traditional Nursing Remedies

Since most traditional mothers nursed, special foods were also encouraged to create more milk. Filipinas recommend bitter foods, such as bitter fish stew, to increase a mother's milk. One Chinese-American says that her mother made her pig's feet stewed with raw peanuts. My mother suggested hard-boiled eggs cooked in sweet black vinegar boiled with ginger. After the twelfth day, she says, you can add pig's feet. Korean-Americans swear by their seaweed soup to increase milk production, along with meat soup with bones, and milk. Taboo foods include spicy and salty foods; medicine; beverages and foods containing caffeine; bulgur; and ginseng. The Japanese eat fresh figs, *mochi* (sweetened, sticky rice cake), cooked pumpkin, or soup stock made from koi fish. Even better, drink the blood of the koi fish!

If these foods give you too much milk, my aunt, a Singapore ob/gyn, suggests putting some chilled cabbage leaves on your breasts. Discard the leaves when they lose their cold. But don't do this too long, she says; your milk will dry up.

For sore nipples, Western doctors recommend exposing them to air so they dry and using ointments such as A&D lotion or breast milk to lubricate them. Or try this: My friend's Japanese grandmother suggests putting fish scales on the nipples to cool the fever.

If you're worried about how to cook any of the special

postpartum foods or remedies, take a tip from the Malaysian-Chinese: They hire a special maid called *phui yuet* for the month at a cost of $700, just to look after the mother and child. She cooks five meals a day for the mother, and does the mother's wash. A note to the dads: Fathers and other family members must fend for themselves!

A Charmed Life: Caring for Your New Baby

While family members and maids are looking after the mother, the mother is looking after her new child. In traditional times, the care was constant, around-the-clock. In Japan, for example, the child was bundled on her mother's back, held by a broad band of cloth wrapped around the baby's bottom and her back. There the child would remain all day, sleeping and waking when she pleased. If the mother wasn't holding the baby, an older sister might take a turn. The baby stayed in direct physical contact with her parents even at night, when the family bed was the norm.

Other baby practices include a solution for a misshapen head. A baby's skull bones are very soft. When a baby favors one side when sleeping, the head may become flatter on that side. Western doctors advise mothers to alternate the side on which the baby sleeps. The Chinese fill a baby's pillow with rice or beans to make it hard, believing that only then will the head have the proper shape.

To encourage a strong step, Chinese mothers once bound their child's ankles loosely with a wide ribbon to keep the feet in an upright position. Then, it was believed, the child would walk with feet pointing forward, not too far to the side.

Protecting Your Child from Evil Spirits

Just as important as the child's physical day-to-day care was the child's protection from the many evil spirits and otherworldly gods who might cause mischief. In the days when infant mortality was high, it was believed that a child died because the gods stole him away. Many rituals and sacred charms were used to shield the baby from their whims. In China and Japan, for example, it is believed that some demons use small children to reinforce the foundations of bridges. As an antidote, mothers and fathers fashion arrows from the wood of the peach tree to place near the cradle. Golden bells tied on the wrists and ankles of children are also used to keep away the bad spirits. In Southern China, a charm is pinned onto a pair of the father's trousers and placed near the cradle. The hope is that the spirit will be attracted by the charm and miss the child.

Nervous or timid children were thought to be so because they could see evil spirits that others could not. To protect these children, Chinese mothers placed small amounts of vermilion in red pouches. The pouches were attached to the children's clothing and were supposed to make them unafraid.

Some amulets, like the Western rabbit's foot, are Asian-variety good luck charms. The Chinese tie coins together with a red string to wear as an amulet for a rich, healthy life. Cradles in Japan are made from peach wood—peach is the symbol for immortality, and so is a wish for a long life—or pine, a wish for an admirable life.

Even the baby's clothing has tiny charms sewn on, wishes for wealth or protection against evil. A Chinese cap may have symbols of happiness and long life embroidered on it. Coins symbolize wealth and family status; the intricate needlework is meant to attract only friendly spirits. A baby girl in Korea may have shiny metal ornaments braided into her hair to deflect the spirits who may cause illness. Earrings may be placed in the ears of boy babies to disguise them as girls. (The spirits, we are told, prefer boys.) When a Chinese baby is especially frail, the parents may ask friends for bits of cloth to sew into a patchwork coat. This disguises the child as a poor child whom the evil spirits need not disturb. And during times of epidemics or contagious illnesses, Chinese mothers protect their children by stitching pieces of red cloth to their clothing.

Baby shoes also carry significance. In China, a young boy's tiny shoes may display fanciful embroidered tigers. Tigers are the bearer of the male principle, the ruler of the animal kingdom, protector against demons. The red lining on the inside is the symbol of life and good fortune. A Korean child's booties are always too large for her small feet, a subtle wish for her growth and long life.

Some parents went to great lengths to protect their children from gods or ghosts who may have harmed them. One turn-of-the-century missionary in China reported seeing young boys dressed in the attire of Buddhist priests. Their parents, fearing for their lives, took them to the local temples, where they were dedicated to enter the priesthood. These boys continued to live at home. At the age of thirteen or fifteen, their fathers returned the child to the temple, bringing with them a bench, a package of chopsticks, a broom, and a dustpan. The priest then asked the child to sweep the floor and clean the walls. Pretending not to be satisfied with his work, the priest would order the child to leave the temple, telling him he was not wanted. The child would jump over the bench—symbolizing the walls of the temple—and the priest would throw the chopsticks after him. He would run all the way home, never looking back, and thus was freed from his religious vow.

That's an extreme case. But don't we all have these deep fears and desires as parents—fervent, prayerful hopes that our children will grow and prosper? In the dark of night, how many times have we called upon the gods to protect our precious charges from the chances of life? How many times have we gazed upon the peaceful innocence of our children, or comforted a sobbing child, or kissed a grazed knee, and wished that we could forever shield them? As parents, new or old, we join the generations of parents before us who tried in every way they knew to take care of their children. The rituals such as sitting the month, the superstitions, the amulets, the special herbs and foods may seem strange to our Western-tuned ears. But in the heart and soul of these rites are the same promptings and wishes and powerful love that we feel today. Baby TV monitors, fire-retardant clothing, cribs that conform to federal standards, triangle bumpers intended to prevent SIDS—these are our new, modern-day amulets. Perhaps all we really need are tiger-faced booties.

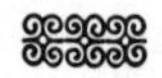

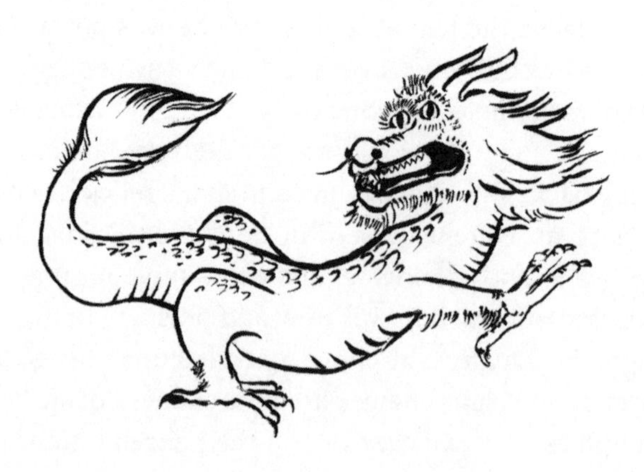

7

Celebrations

I cannot tell all the ceremonies that followed in the days and months after my daughter's birth. I would tire of the telling, there are so many. There was the feast to celebrate the girl's first bath; magic parcels hung by my door to give her good character; and demon-catchers surrounded me and my child . . .

RITUALS OF BIRTH, CHINA, 1860

THE BIRTH OF A CHILD IS THE CAUSE OF CELEBRATION in every culture. Here in the West, we have baby showers, christenings, briths. Friends and family visit to ooh and ahh over the tiny hands, the perfect feet. Cards, flowers, and more gifts are received. But few cultures have as elaborate, as mysterious, or as symbolic baby celebrations as the Asians. In the first hundred days of a Chinese baby's life, for example, she stars at no fewer than five events celebrating her tiny life.

At each event, there is a mix of spiritual and practical rites. There are offerings to placate the gods and announce to the ancestors the baby's entrance into the family. There are delicious, home-cooked foods for Mom to replenish her strength. There are an abundance of baby gifts, gold jewelry, silver toys, and fancifully embroidered clothes. At every turn, the family gathers to give thanks for the health of the child and offers prayers for the baby's continued growth, his future prosperity, her good fortune.

Many Asian-Americans have brought these rituals to their new homes in America. If they're not followed to the letter, perhaps a Japanese grandparent may say special prayers on the baby's thirty-second day of life, or a Chinese auntie may offer the traditional red envelope full of shiny gold coins. Rituals vary from village to village, family to family. Ask your relatives what traditions heralded your arrival, or their own births. You may even want to add some Asian touches to your Western-style baby celebrations. Serving red-dyed, hardboiled eggs or Korean rice cakes at your baby shower, or giving small sets of silver chopsticks, might be a fun way to honor your baby's ancestry and make the event special.

There are many cultural and family traditions that celebrate a baby's coming. Here are a few of the more well-known Asian traditions celebrated, from the third day to the child's first steps:

THIRD DAY

On the morning of the third day, a Chinese baby gets his or her first bath. The midwife who was present at the birth usually officiates at this ceremony, which is attended by mostly women friends and relatives. The midwife sits with the mother on her bed (remember, the mother is still sitting the month and cannot leave the room), surrounded by a straw sieve, a mirror, a padlock, an onion, a comb, and a weight. An offering of incense to the god and goddess of the bed burns nearby.

Hot water boiled with locust branches—as a disinfectant, and artemis plants—for perfume, is poured into a large metal basin. Around the basin are a piece of red silk and a string of cash. The friends then enter the room, greeting the mother and offering congratulations. Each guest then places a piece of fruit or some nuts and a colored egg (two if it's a girl) into the water. White eggs are a wish for long life; the white symbolizes the white hair of the aged. Red eggs are used as a wish for luck. Each guest also places a spoonful of cool water into the basin, and a small silver gift on the bed. The cool water is symbolic: The word for "cool," *shui,* also sounds like the word for "clever," a wish that the child will grow to be smart. Now the baby is ready for her first bath.

In olden times, the midwife might stir the bathwater as she bathed the baby, chanting:

I chiao, er chiao, lien san chiao,
Ko ko ken chih titi pa'o

Once stirred, twice stirred, thrice altogether.
Big brother is here, a younger comes hither.

In some areas, a slice of green ginger may be rubbed against the baby's navel during the bath to charm away sickness.

After the bath is finished, the baby is wrapped in a towel and dried. The midwife then takes up the items on the bed. The weight is placed on the child, and the midwife chants:

Ch'eng t'o hsiao yu ch'ien chin.

The weight might be small,
but it is as heavy as one thousand pounds.

The superstitious believe that a child who dies is running away from the earth. The weight is supposed to weigh the child down to prevent escape. The onion—its name sounds like the word for "clever"—is tapped on the baby as a wish that the baby will grow to be smart. The midwife may say these lines:

I ta ts'ung ming. Er ta kung ming.

Once touched and wisdom came.
Twice touched and great was his fame.

The onion is then thrown over the house so it's not used again.

The padlock is held over the body and snapped shut, locking the child to this world. While pretending to comb the baby's hair, the midwife says,

San shu tzu, liang lung tzu.
Chang ta la, tai hung ting tzu.

Thrice comb, twice comb, carefully comb the hair
And when he is grown, a red button he will wear.

The red button is a reference to the button worn by high officials in China's history.

Next, the baby is held over the sieve while it is shaken. It was once believed that smallpox, called by the Chinese "flower from heaven," would fall from above, pass through the sieve, and never harm the child. His first vaccination!

Last, the midwife goes to the next room, where offerings were made to Niang Niang, the goddess of childbirth. The paper pictures of the goddess are gathered and burned, along with the pictures of the god and goddess of the bed. The midwife ties a small amount of these ashes in red silk, which is then sewn to the baby's pillow to protect the baby from evil.

The mother also receives gifts on the third day, mostly food to bolster her strength. Chickens, sweetmeats, uncooked eggs, and red-colored eggs are given. The red color in this instance symbolizes joy.

Seventh Day—*Oshichiya*, "Seven Evenings"

On the seventh day of life, a Japanese child receives its name in a ceremony organized by the midwife. Family and friends gather to congratulate the new arrival, and presents are brought for both mother and child.

Twelfth Day

On this day, the Chinese mother's mother brings her food—sometimes meat dumplings—to help her get strong. She is now allowed to walk around in her room, though because of her confinement, she is not permitted to walk farther than the courtyard.

In Malaysia, the new mother receives her first bath since the delivery on this day. Herbs are added to purify the water, which must be boiled.

Twenty-ninth/Thirtieth Days

On the twenty-ninth day, a Chinese boy gets his head shaved; a girl is shaved on the thirtieth day. The hair that is shaved is wrapped in a piece of red cloth and sewn to the end of the baby's pillow. When the child is a hundred days old, the hair is thrown into a river or lake to ensure that the child will be brave and fearless.

My mother offers another reason to shave the baby's

head: She says her family believes that the hair will grow thicker if it is shaved. Also, the fine hair of babies always falls out on its own in the first few months. Shaving the head stops the hair from falling out and reduces the amount that the baby involuntarily swallows.

One Month—
Man Yueh

The biggest celebration for the Chinese newborn is at one month. The mother is finally allowed out of her room, and family and friends are invited to dine and party all night. The house is decorated with flowers and with large banners decorated with the character for "joy." In wealthier families of long ago, theater groups were invited to perform; one party had a marionette show running throughout the party for parents and children alike!

More presents are given to the little one. These may include clothing, including shoes and caps, silver ornaments, and silk. Money is given in bright red envelopes. Nine idols are fastened on the baby's cap for luck, and around his or her neck, the baby wears a silver or gold padlock on a red string, "locking" the child to this world. If the baby is born to a family who recently lost a child, a special charm called *po chia so,* a hundred-person lock, is placed on the padlock. This lock is purchased with the coins from a hundred friends whose names may even be inscribed on a gold pendant suspended from the lock.

Thus, with so many well-wishers, the child has even more reason to stay!

Among the rural Chinese in Malaysia, it is the friends of the father who are invited to the one-month celebration. Festivities include the shaving of the baby's head. At that time, an empty green coconut is placed in a brass pan filled with water. A female relative shaves the baby's head and places the hair into the coconut. The coconut is then thrown into the sea.

THIRTY-TWO/THIRTY-THREE DAYS— *MIYA MAIRI*, "SHRINE VISITING"

On the thirty-second day for a boy, the thirty-third day for a girl, the Japanese newborn is taken to the Shinto shrine or to the *ujigami*, the tutelary shrine of the family, to be introduced to the gods. The ceremony, which is much like a baptism, is organized by the midwife and performed by a Shinto priest. For the occasion, the child is dressed in a formal kimono for the first time. Like a baptism, *miya mairi* allows the child to participate in other religious events at the temple.

ONE-HUNDRED-DAY CELEBRATION— *PAIK IL*

In Korea, the biggest celebration for the newborn is held after a hundred days, at the *paik il*. At this time, the infant is no longer deemed fragile. The parents are now more certain that the baby will live, and they celebrate the occasion. One party or several may be held, depending on the family. It is a large party, with lots of food and delicacies such as *dok,* a special Korean rice cake. At this time, even more gifts are given, such as a set of silver chopsticks, a silver spoon, a gold baby ring, or clothing. (Most Koreans wait until the *paik il* to give baby gifts.) Traditionally, invitations to this event were sent with a plate of rice cakes and other delicacies.

If you're invited to a *paik il,* or decide to hold one of your own, teach your friends the Korean words for "congratulations": *"Paik il ul chook ha ha hahm ni da."*

One interesting side note: A studio photograph is taken on this day to commemorate the event. Traditionally, boys are photographed naked to show off their prized "pepper." Girls, however, are photographed fully clothed.

The Chinese also have some traditions for the hundredth day. On that day, friends and relatives take presents of fish and chicken to the house. When the chicken is cooked, the tongue is pulled out and rubbed on the lips of the baby. This is a wish that the child will be a good talker. And traditionally, the baby's paternal grandfather also presents him or her with the gift of a rocking chair on this day.

109 Days—*Tabezome*

Tabezome, held 109 days after birth, celebrates the Japanese baby's first intake of solid food. A small table with a bowl of boiled rice, rice paste, or soup is prepared for the baby. Chopsticks—red and black for a girl, black for a boy—are placed next to the bowl. The mother kneels before the table and, with baby in lap, feeds a single grain of rice to her child. Family and friends are usually on hand to witness this important event, which in olden times marked the baby's acceptance into the community.

First Birthday

The Chinese child's first birthday is celebrated with a great feast, and offerings to the gods and ancestors. The maternal grandmother is again the major gift-giver, bestowing more clothes and food on her grandchild. The food consists of chicken—some families rub a chicken's tongue over the child's lips at the first birthday—and prawns so that the child will learn to catch herself if she falls, much as a prawn uses its claws. A long bread, *yu char kuei,* usually eaten at breakfast, is also given to the child for the first time. According to the old wives' tale, eating this bread will help him learn to walk.

The main tradition is a game in which a variety of objects are placed in a basket before the child: a pen, ink, ink slab, silver, an official seal, needlework, a flower, and some toys. Whatever the child grabs first indicates what he'll be later in life. If he grabs a pen or the ink, he'll be a scholar. If he reaches for the silver, he'll be wealthy. If he grabs the flower or the toys, he'll be a society rogue and not amount to much of anything. If the child is a girl, according to tradition, she'll marry someone with these traits.

This is a fun game to play on a first birthday, when the highlight is usually watching cake get smeared around the baby's face or keeping wrapping paper out of his mouth. We played this game on my son's first birthday but altered it a bit to reflect more modern and American ways. We piled all sorts of items on a tray—a bottle of medicine (for a doctor), a gavel (for a lawyer), a train (for an engineer), toys, a shiny pen, and a pile of coins. He chose the medicine. My son, the doctor!

In Korea, the first birthday, or *ddol,* is celebrated with even more festivities, more panache, than the hundred-day celebration. In fact, it is one of the two important birthdays marked in the lives of most Koreans: the first and the sixtieth. On this day, children are dressed in traditional Korean costume: baggy silk trousers, shirt, vest, and jacket for the boys; a long skirt and short top with long, rounded sleeves for the girls. Both also wear a black hat decorated with gold trim.

The traditional first-birthday gift is a gold ring. This harkens back to the times when the rings were meant as an insurance against hard times. Gold could always be sold for cash in times of famine or illness.

The best part of the Korean first birthday is the meal, *tolsang*. Traditionally, the celebration was held during breakfast time, but now that most people work and live in cities, it is held in the evening. It is a true feast. There may be platters of noodles, fruits and cookies, and rice. Dishes are set out on a traditional low table with other symbolic items such as a writing brush and ink stone, book, cotton thread, money, and an archery bow, to wish the child luck and success. Besides the *dok,* the rice cake served at all important events, *moo jee gae dok,* or rainbow *dok,* is presented. Made from sweetened, chewy rice, the cake has layers of pink, green, brown, and white. Steamed rice cakes, millet dumplings, and stuffed jujube fruits may also be served.

First Steps

There are few moments more exciting during the first year of a baby's life than when she takes her first steps. Videocamera rolling, you jump up and down while those wobbling legs move forward and the child grins a toothy smile.

But if you're of Chinese ancestry, be sure to cut the cord that binds your child to the nether world. The Chinese believe that around the ankles of your child are invisible bindings that tie her to her previous life. When a child takes her first steps, a relative walks behind her with a knife and draws three lines on the ground. Then, with the bindings cut, she will walk freely forever.

As your baby grows, there are so many uniquely Asian ways to celebrate childhood. For those of Chinese or Korean background, there are kite-flying days in spring and at New Year's. The Chinese celebrate New Year's, too, with special lantern parades for the children and a wild dragon dance. For a Japanese-American child there is Girls' Day on March 3, and Boys' Festival on May 5. And a special day for children with gifts and outings is celebrated in Korea on May 5. As your child grows, one foot in this land, one foot in a culture that can seem strange and foreign, you may wish to take advantage of these special times. Like the celebrations and rituals of childbirth, they are a time to gather the family together, to define what family means, to show love and appreciation to each other. For children with many different backgrounds, these celebrations can help form bridges to grandparents who don't speak English, or have different customs. Or they can simply help these multicultural and diverse flowers feel the beauty within themselves. No matter what you choose to do, celebrate the precious gift of life you have been blessed with, and enjoy each step of the way.

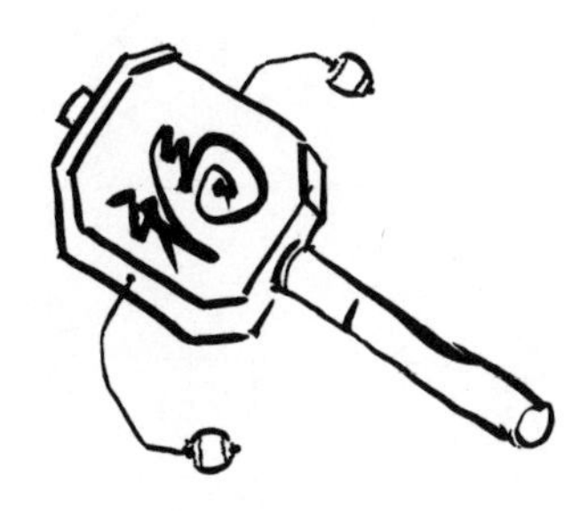

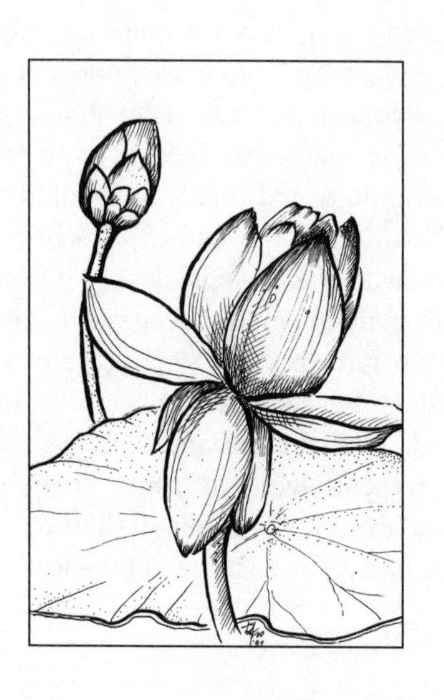

8

Nursery Rhymes, Stories, and Songs

OUR BABY

Mrs. Chang, Mrs. Lee,
Mama has a small baby;
stands up firm,
sits up straight,
won't eat milk,
but lives on cake.

EVERY LANGUAGE AND CULTURE has its own special way of speaking to its littlest members. No matter where you travel, you'll find mothers and fathers crooning to their babies in the sweetest of voices. The words may be unfamiliar—not every song will sound like "Twinkle, Twinkle," not every rhyme like "Little Boy Blue." But the love, the gentle murmur of the melody, the security and caress of well-worn rhythms, are the same.

These pieces of literature I've found come from all over Asia. Some are ancient; some are modern. Many reflect concerns of parents everywhere. Some seem particular to the culture they originate from. Others, like many of the Mother Goose rhymes, have dark sentiments of hardship and illness—perhaps a reflection of the struggles of humanity's youngest members. Others are full of the simple innocence of childhood. Enjoy them. And be sure to ask your own parents and grandparents for some gems of their own.

JAPANESE LULLABY

Sleep, sleep.
Be a good child and sleep.
Your Nan went over the mountains
to reach her village.

When she comes back
she will bring you drums
and flutes as a gift to you,
and with these toys
she will bring you to sleep.

Typical traditional Vietnamese lullabies often include cooking tips and moral tales.

VIETNAMESE LULLABY

To make a soup of fish and pumpkin
add some pepper and chives to bring out the taste.
Sleep soundly, my baby,
so I can work to feed you.

The bridge is made of nailed planks,
and crossing a rickety bamboo bridge is most difficult of all.

CHINESE LULLABY

Hsiao hai tzu
Kuai shui chiao
Ming tien tai ni
Chu kuang miao.

Little baby mine,
sleep, sleep fast.
Tomorrow I'll take thee
to a temple vast.

Songs

It's true, music *is* the universal language. From Europe to Asia to Africa, children's songs from all around the world seem to have similar themes. Here are two from China about the boogeyman:

Feng lai la
Yu lai la
Lao he hsang pei chih
Ku lai la.

Wind is blowing,
rain is falling.
The old man comes,
his thunder calling.

GO TO SLEEP

The tree leaves are murmuring hua-la-la;
Baby's very sleepy and wants his mama.
Go to sleep, my baby, and then go to bed,
and any boogey-boo that comes,
I'll knock him on the head.

Even pat-a-cake is common in all cultures. Here's the Chinese version:

Kuang, kuang cha
Kuang, kuang cha
Miao li he shang
Mei yu tou fa.

Cymbals a pair,
cymbals a pair.
The old temple priest,
he has no hair.

And doesn't this verse from China sound like something from Mother Goose?

Hung ku lu chiao che
Pai ma la
Li tou tsorh chih I ko
Chiao jen chia
Hui shu, piao yin shu kua
Tui tzu ho pao

Hsiao chihrh cha
Pa chih che yuan rh
Wen a ko, "A ko, a ko ni shang narh?"

"Wo tao nan pien'rh
Chiao ching chia,
Chiao wan ching chia,
Tao wo chia"

"Ta tzu po-po, chui nai cha
Chih wan la, wo sung ni hui chia."

Inside a red-wheeled cart,
white horse–drawn,
sits a man dressed so smart,
all alone.

Fur coat of gray, fur coat of white,
with a pair of gay bags
sewed in colors bright.

Lean on the shafts, look inside;
ask this man where he goes:

"I go South,
my friends to see."

"When you adjourn,
come see me.
I'll give you cake, milk, and tea
before you return."

Here's a song from China that my parents taught my son when he was one. He still sings it, though he is the only one who knows all the words!

YEH LIANG AH
(O MOON!)

Yeh liang ah,
Yeh liang ah!
Wo ai ni.
Lai, lai, lai—
Chin ni chong tian shan xia lai.
Lai, lai, lai—
Chin ni chong tian shan xia lai.

Xiao ti-ti,
Xiao mae-mae,
Wo pu nan cau xia lai.
Wo pu nan cau xia lai.

O Moon,
O Moon!
I love you.
Come, come, come—
Please come down from heaven.

Little brother,
little sister,
I cannot come down from heaven.
I cannot come down from heaven.

Here's another song from China:

I-KEN TZU CHU CHIH MIAO-MIAO (PURPLE STRAIGHT-GROWN BAMBOO SHOOT)

I-ken tzu chu chih miao-miao
Sung yu bao-bao tso kuan hsiao.
Hsiao-erh tui cheng k'ou
K'ou-erh tui cheng hsiao.
Hsiao chung ch'ui ch'u shih hsin tiao,
Hsiao bao-bao,
U-ti, u-ti,
Hsueh hui liao!

Purple straight-grown bamboo shoot,
to my pet sent for a flute.
Put it to your lips,
lips to the flute.
From the flute new music comes,
little treasure.
Eetee, eetee—
You've learned how!

The following nursery rhymes were first collected in 1900 under the title *Chinese Mother Goose Rhymes.* The translator, Isaac Taylor Headland of Peking University, said in his original preface: "There are probably more nursery rhymes in China than can be found in England and

America. . . . There is no language in the world, we venture to believe, which contains children's songs expressive of more keen and tender affection than [these]." I find them fascinating for their glimpse into a child's life of long ago.

You can find these and other nursery rhymes in a book now entitled *Chinese Nursery Rhymes,* published by W. M. Hawley Publications of Hollywood, California.

COME AND PLAY

Little baby, full of glee,
won't you come and play with me?
And at the picnic place we'll call.
And you shall come and drink my tea.
When I invite you thus to play?
How is it that you run away?

CHICKEN SKIN

I went ten steps outside the gate,
which brought me to the ditches,
and there I found some chicken skin
to mend my leather breeches;
if there had been no chicken skin,
I could not mend my trousers thin.

GO TO BED

Little baby, go to bed,
we'll put a hoop around your head,

and with the oil we get thereby,
our little bean-cake we will fry.

And when we've fried our bean-cake brown,
we'll see the king go into town,
an iron cap upon his head;
now you must surely go to bed.

GRANDPA FEEDS BABY

Grandpa holds the baby,
he's sitting on his knee.
Eating mutton dumplings
with vinegar and tea.
Then grandpa says to baby,
"When you have had enough,
you'll be a saucy baby
and treat your grandpa rough."

LITTLE SMALL-FEET

The small-footed girl
with the sweet little smile,
she loves to eat sugar
and sweets all the while.
Her money's all gone
and because she can't buy,
she holds her small feet
while she sits down to cry.

THE LITTLE ORPHAN

Like a withered flower,
that is dying in the earth,
I am left alone at seven,
by her who gave me birth.

With my papa I was happy,
but I feared he'd take another,
and now my papa's married,
and I have a little brother.

And he eats good food,
while I eat poor,
and cry for my mother,
whom I see no more.

BABY IS SLEEPING

My baby is sleeping,
my baby's asleep,
my flower is resting,
I'll give you a peep;
how cunning he looks
as he rests on my arm!
My flower's most charming
of all them that charm.

LITTLE FAT BOY

What a bonnie fellow is this fat boy of mine!
He makes people die of joy!
What a fine little fellow is this fat boy of mine!
Now whose is this loving little boy?

Do you want to buy a beauty?
Do you want to buy a beauty?
If you buy him he will watch your house,
and do it as his duty.

And no matter as to servants,
you may have them or may not,
but you'll never need to lock your door
or give your house a thought.

POUNDING RICE

Pound, pound,
pound the rice.
The pestle goes up and down so nice.
Open the pot,
the fire is hot,
and if you don't eat
I'll feed you rice.

Tales of the Moon

The moon has always been a source of much folklore in Asia. When I was growing up, my father told me not about the man in the moon, but about the rabbit that circled round and round it. When the moon is full, you can actually see the rabbit, his ears streaming behind him as he circles round the moon. According to legend, the rabbit adorns the moon because of his devotion to Buddha. One day, Buddha asked for some food and water from his followers. All the animals searched high and low for the choicest morsels for the Buddha. The rabbit, however, embarrassed by his offerings of grass and herbs, leaped into the fire to offer up the best meal he could: himself.

As a reward, the rabbit pounds the elixir of immortality under a grove of cassia trees on the moon. On clear nights, parents point toward the moon and tell this story of devotion and sacrifice. Perhaps you might tell your children, too.

Korea's famous moon tale is about a loving brother and sister who lived with their mother. When she was coming home from market one day, a tiger attacked her at a mountain pass and ate her. Like the big bad wolf in the story of Red Riding Hood, the tiger went to her house disguised as the mother and called out for the boy and girl. But the brother and sister were smarter than that; they knew the voice came from a dreadful tiger.

The two ran as fast as they could to the top of a tall tree. As the tiger began to climb the tree, they prayed to God to protect them. God saved them and brought them to heaven, where the boy became the sun and the girl the moon.

In Japan, they tell the tale of a bamboo cutter who found a baby in a bamboo stem. He and his wife raised the baby girl as their own, calling her Kaguyahime, the Shining Princess. She grew up to be as beautiful as her name, and was courted by wealthy and powerful suitors, including the Emperor himself. She eluded them all, however, by asking that they perform impossible deeds to win her hand.

Finally, she explained to her earthly parents that she was from the palace on the moon, and that she had to return there. Sadly, she departed. But each full moon, Japanese children can pick out the outlines of Kaguyahime's lunar palace in the sky.

One of the most popular inhabitants of the moon in Chinese folklore is the goddess Chang E. Her husband, Hou Yi, is known as the master archer of the skies. One day, ten suns appeared in the sky and threatened life on earth. Hou Yi took out his bow and arrows and shot down nine of the ten suns. As a reward, the Queen Mother of the West gave him the elixir of life.

Chang E found this magic potion and drank it up. She

began to rise, and flew all the way to the moon, where she turned into a three-legged toad. From that day, Chang E has ruled over the lunar kingdom, while her husband rules over the solar kingdom. They meet once a month on the fifteenth day, when the moon is full.

At the Moon Festival in mid-September, when the harvest moon is at its brightest, children dress in fancy clothes and make secret wishes to Chang E, goddess of the moon.

Momotaro, the Peach Boy

This last tale is remembered by many Japanese, even those who have grown up on these shores. It is a true fairy tale, as heroic and magical as any we've grown up with in the West. I hope you pass it along to your children.

Once upon a time, an old woodcutter and his wife lived at the edge of the forest in a distant province in Japan. Though they loved children, they were yet to be blessed with one. As the years went by without a child, they grew sadder and sadder. But they never gave up hope, and continued to offer their prayers and sacrifices to the gods.

One day, the woodcutter's wife went to a stream nearby to do some washing. Bobbing on the surface was the biggest, most beautiful, most delectable peach she had ever seen. She grabbed it and carried it joyfully home. It was so large and so splendid that she and her husband hardly dared to cut it open.

As soon as the knife touched the skin of the peach, out jumped a baby boy, with skin golden and pink like a peach and a nature even sweeter. Surely he was a gift from the gods. And so, they named him Momotaro, Son of the Peach.

Momotaro grew up to be handsome and kind and sweet. When he was grown, he told his mother and father that he had to prove himself to the world. With a bag of rice dumplings his mother made him and a sword given to him by his father, he set out far beyond his village to the terrible Oni Island.

The oni are ugly, horrible monsters, tall as pine trees, with horns like demons and tusks like elephants. Their bodies are colored deep red, blue, green, and black, as black as their deeds. For generations, they had terrified the countryside, killing all in their path and stealing some of Japan's most precious treasure.

On his way to Oni Island, Momotaro met three friends: the Lord Dog, the Lord Monkey, and the Lord Pheasant. Each one pledged his solidarity to Momotaro and his quest, and to each he gave a dumpling. "One dumpling," he said to them, "will give you the strength of ten men."

The four brave travelers reached the shore, found a boat, and rowed across the deep sea to Oni Island. There they could see the gloomy fortress of Oni Castle and hear the sounds of a wild feast. For a moment they were afraid, but the dumplings had given them the strength of thousands of men, and they plotted their attack.

Lord Monkey climbed to the top of the wall, the Lord Pheasant flew to the gatepost, and Lord Dog hid behind the gate. Momotaro banged loudly at the door. A big red oni answered.

"Who are you?" he growled, angry at being disturbed.

"I am Momotaro," Momotaro replied, "and I've come to conquer you."

The oni threw back his head and laughed a horrible, ground-shaking laugh, and called his friends over to see the funny human who thought he could conquer them. Soon thousands of oni came out to see the fuss. But as they came lumbering through the gates, Lord Pheasant pecked out their eyes, and Lord Monkey twisted their necks. Lord Dog knocked them down, and Momotaro finished them off with the sword his father had given him.

When three thousand oni had been killed, the leader surrendered, begging forgiveness. In return for his pardon, he returned Japan's treasure and promised never to do evil again. When the Emperor heard of the noble deed of Momotaro and his friends, he granted them a reward and declared a day of thanksgiving. They returned to the woodcutter and his wife, who were overjoyed to see them. They all lived together happily for the rest of their lives, and Japan never saw another oni again.

Conclusion: A New Beginning

MY SECOND SON WAS BORN just as this book was completed, just a few short weeks ago. He grew within me as these pages took shape, with thoughts of my ancestors and their lucky stars, with birth dreams of my very own. It seems only fitting that he made his entrance into this world as these stories came to life—"You've had two births," someone said to me.

I never did get to crush ginger in the doorway to ease the labor, but, perhaps in his eagerness to see the world, my son made it easy for me anyway. With a patch of black hair and dancing, dark eyes, he came screaming into the world, but calmed down as my husband and I whispered prayers in his ears. We named him Chad Yeh—Yeh to follow in the footsteps of his wonderful big brother, Keith Yeh, and the rest of his generation. Born in the year of the Ox, he is a content child, peaceful and happy. In these first few days of his life, my husband and I often catch ourselves staring at the bounty of our family, shaking our heads in wonderment at our two sons. The gods were kind once more, and we feel so very blessed.

With my mother's and father's help, I did "sit the month." I did it American-style: I ate the right foods, but did shower and wash my hair. Looking back on those first few weeks, I realize a bit of this tradition's ageless wisdom. My month, in the waning days of a beautiful summer, was a priceless time. Freed from life's busy schedule, I was able to take the time to welcome and learn about my new son; to take the time to cherish my first son, to feel cocooned within the arms of my family, new and old, to heal and gain my strength—physical and spiritual—for the days ahead.

I am a different mother today than I was when Keith was born. Among other things, tradition, my ancestry, my heritage, mean more to me. Perhaps when a tree bears fruit, it pays more attention to its deepest roots. Perhaps enshrined in these ancient myths are lessons that you see only when they appear at your doorstep, wrapped in a soft baby blanket.

My children, like your children, will grow in two worlds, one Asian, one American. I want them to wonder at the rabbit who runs around the moon, to thrill at the heart-thumps of a dragon dance, to chase after the dancing tail of a kite soaring on a spring breeze. With the myths and the stories of the ancients in their hearts, I want them to embrace this life comfortable in their unique heritage, ready to give their own special gifts to this world.

. . . But that is to come. Right now, I want to treasure this time, with Chad cradled in my arms and Keith growing tall beside me. A lotus pod, with its many seeds, can last forever; childhood lasts but a moment. In a few days, we will celebrate Chad's *man yueh,* whole month, with traditional foods, close family, and good friends. It is a celebration of life, a life given, a life blessed. I hope it will be long and full of love. And I wish the same for you.

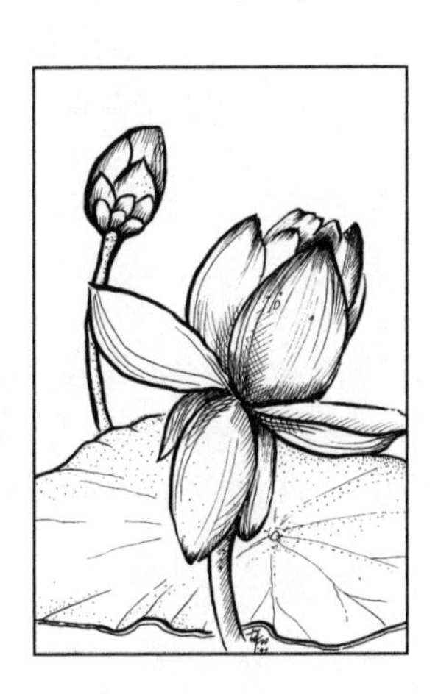